Setting Limits
Gambling, Science, and
Public Policy

T0323395

Setting Limits
Gambling, Science, and Public Policy

Pekka Sulkunen, Thomas F. Babor,
Jenny Cisneros Örnberg, Michael Egerer,
Matilda Hellman, Charles Livingstone,
Virve Marionneau, Janne Nikkinen,
Jim Orford, Robin Room, and
Ingeborg Rossow

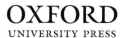

OXFORD
UNIVERSITY PRESS

OXFORD
UNIVERSITY PRESS

Great Clarendon Street, Oxford, OX2 6DP,
United Kingdom

Oxford University Press is a department of the University of Oxford.
It furthers the University's objective of excellence in research, scholarship,
and education by publishing worldwide. Oxford is a registered trade mark of
Oxford University Press in the UK and in certain other countries

© Oxford University Press 2019

The moral rights of the authors have been asserted

First Edition published in 2019

Impression: 1

All rights reserved. No part of this publication may be reproduced, stored in
a retrieval system, or transmitted, in any form or by any means, without the
prior permission in writing of Oxford University Press, or as expressly permitted
by law, by licence or under terms agreed with the appropriate reprographics
rights organization. Enquiries concerning reproduction outside the scope of the
above should be sent to the Rights Department, Oxford University Press, at the
address above

You must not circulate this work in any other form
and you must impose this same condition on any acquirer

Published in the United States of America by Oxford University Press
198 Madison Avenue, New York, NY 10016, United States of America

British Library Cataloguing in Publication Data

Data available

Library of Congress Control Number: 2018945619

ISBN 978–0–19–881732–1

Printed and bound by
CPI Group (UK) Ltd, Croydon, CR0 4YY

Oxford University Press makes no representation, express or implied, that the
drug dosages in this book are correct. Readers must therefore always check
the product information and clinical procedures with the most up-to-date
published product information and data sheets provided by the manufacturers
and the most recent codes of conduct and safety regulations. The authors and
the publishers do not accept responsibility or legal liability for any errors in the
text or for the misuse or misapplication of material in this work. Except where
otherwise stated, drug dosages and recommendations are for the non-pregnant
adult who is not breast-feeding

Links to third party websites are provided by Oxford in good faith and
for information only. Oxford disclaims any responsibility for the materials
contained in any third party website referenced in this work.

Foreword

Different types of gambling have been known for centuries and attempts to regulate gambling can also be found throughout the history of human societies. The nature and dramatic consequences of non-controlled, pathological or compulsive gambling have been described in literature, sometimes, as in the case of Fyodor Dostoevsky and his "The Gambler", based on the author's personal experience. Since the ninth revision of the *International Classification of Diseases* (ICD) (1975) "pathological gambling" has been included in the list of mental and behavioural disorders, and in ICD-9 "gambling and betting" was listed among lifestyle risk factors to health. Until recently however, gambling has never been considered as an important public health issue that required public health responses to protect the health of individuals and populations.

The book "Setting Limits" authored by an international group of experts, presents, from the public health perspective, a comprehensive assessment of gambling in modern societies. It makes a strong case for public health interventions to protect the health of populations where exposure to gambling, due to commercial factors and technological advances, has increased significantly in some jurisdictions, and has a potential to increase exponentially in others. The observed trend toward bridging the gaming and gambling industries, particularly using advantages offered by online services, can result in unlimited exposure of populations to experiences which can be enjoyable and harmless for many, but cause significant health problems for a few. It is these "few" which are often the most vulnerable and deprived members of society, and their number can add up to millions on the global scale. Do modern societies have a role and an obligation to protect the health of their populations from potential health hazards associated with gambling (or the most risky types of gambling), or does this responsibility have to be left entirely to individuals who decide to be engaged in gambling? Do governments and intergovernmental entities have a role in "consumer protection" from the most hazardous types of gambling and its consequences, or should their role be limited to the support of treatment services for those who develop a gambling disorder? What is the role of health services in prevention of harmful gambling and in treatment for gambling disorder, and what should the funding mechanisms for these prevention and treatment services be? This book provides a wealth of information that can help public health professionals and all those who are interested in public health aspects of gambling to answer these questions.

Public health oriented research on gambling is still at an early stage of development, and the accumulated expertise and available empirical data are largely located in high-income countries. The evidence base for prevention and treatment interventions is very limited, and there is an urgent need to generate data relevant for public health in low- and middle-income countries. Many issues discussed in the book have striking similarities with public health challenges relating to alcohol, tobacco, and psychoactive drug use. In some jurisdictions, regulation of alcohol, drugs, and gambling is overseen by the same areas of government. In the draft 11th revision of the ICD, "gambling disorder" has been moved from the group of "impulse control disorders" to the section of disorders which result from substance use and addictive behaviors. This move is due to the increasing recognition of similarities (although not identity) between these disorders. It is not by coincidence that many authors of this book have an excellent public health record in the area of alcohol and drug policies. There is no doubt that effective and necessary public health measures to minimize public health risks associated with gambling should be based on available evidence of effectiveness of these measures, but also on the lessons learned from other similar areas of public health. "Setting Limits" will serve as an important resource for all stakeholders who see the need for preventing and reducing the public health problems associated with gambling.

Dr Vladimir Poznyak, Coordinator
Management of Substance Abuse
Department of Mental Health and Substance Abuse
World Health Organization, Geneva

Authors' Preface

The idea that led to the publication of this book was conceived over dinner in a traditional Finnish restaurant not far from that country's only gambling casino in Helsinki. In 2012, two of the book's authors (Pekka Sulkunen and Tom Babor) discussed the need for an independent, policy-oriented review of gambling research, and agreed to launch the project by following a successful model used in previous monographs devoted to alcohol and drug policy. The model, consisting of problem-focused integrative literature reviews and epidemiological trend analyses, was first developed by a group of social and behavioral scientists who worked with the World Health Organization on the publication of *Alcohol Control Policies in Public Health Perspective* (Bruun et al. 1975). That book set the stage for subsequent integrative policy reviews (Edwards et al. 1994; Babor et al. 2010) that brought together multidisciplinary groups of scientists to apply public health concepts, methods, and research to address alcohol and drug misuse, long considered to be among the most intractable social problems of modern society.

The question raised at the Finnish restaurant was whether a similar template could be applied to the analysis of gambling problems, which have emerged as a complex social issue that is every bit as challenging as alcohol and drug problems. The challenges to such an endeavor were apparent: a rather sparse scientific literature, the absence of independent funding for the necessary investigative work, and the looming presence of the "Elephant in the Room," the gambling industry.

Despite the expected difficulties in starting this project, the dinner conversation concluded with a handshake and a commitment to find a way to get started. Perhaps it was Lady Luck or the Wheel of Fortune, but the conditions were ripe in Finland and internationally to assemble the necessary resources. First, it helped to have the involvement of the University of Helsinki's Centre for Research on Addiction, Control and Governance. From this resource we were able to quickly assemble a remarkable group of co-authors and research assistants who were capable of tapping into the diverse information sources needed to answer fundamental questions about modern gambling. Second, we were fortunate to engage the financial support of the Finnish Foundation for Alcohol Studies, which generously sponsored several meetings of the investigators as well as the empirical research needed to pursue unanswered questions.

Once the idea had been hatched and funding was secured, the difficult process of writing a multi-authored book was begun. Unlike edited volumes where each author is responsible for a separate chapter, the integrative review of gambling issues we envisioned required authors to produce sections that eventually were synthesized into a meaningful narrative. Although we had an outline that guided our work from the beginning, the themes that constitute the real substance of this book only emerged after the pieces were drafted, discussed, critiqued, re-assembled, and integrated. Three meetings of the co-authors were held to review drafts and discuss emerging themes, and these were interspersed with smaller meetings and collaborations among the co-authors.

The result is a synthesis of ideas, theory, data, and most of all, the world scientific literature devoted to an understanding of gambling, gambling problems, and gambling policy. Authors were required to submerge their egos, their writing styles, and their pet theories into the search for larger meaning in the information we evaluated, to arrive at a view that incorporates the several perspectives held by the participants but nevertheless retains a unique message to policymakers. Authorship of this book is therefore presented in alphabetical order after the two principal authors who coordinated the writing process and integrated the elements produced by the others.

At a time when governments throughout the world are enabling new gambling operations without considering the consequences, what became clear from our review is that the nature of modern gambling, both commercial and government-sponsored, is changing in ways that are likely to exacerbate its negative impact on society and ordinary citizens. In the final analysis, we found that the financial harm, relationship disruption, emotional distress, decrements to health, and socioeconomic inequality are not unintended side-effects of a largely benign recreational activity, but rather the inevitable consequences of bad social policy that is compounded by false beliefs in the ability of treatment, financial counseling, and charity work to cure the ills that gambling creates.

Far from the idealized story of the novice gambler who hits the jackpot and lives happily ever after, the message from our review is that in modern gambling the deck is stacked in favor of the house, with most people paying dearly for a game where the odds are always against them. If this book helps to shift the policy perspective to preventing the corporate and political winners from taking advantage of those who can least afford it, it will have proven to be a winning bet.

Acknowledgements

The main sponsor of this project was the Finnish Foundation for Alcohol Studies. The authors are particularly grateful to the Foundation for its support for the work conducted by Pekka Sulkunen and the sponsorship of three meetings of the authors. Most of all, we appreciate the encouragement provided by the Foundation's Research Director, Tomi Lintonen, who gave the authors complete freedom to speak with an independent voice in the interest of effective gambling policy. The Academy of Finland has provided resources for original research that we have conducted to fill gaps in the existing science. A research centre grant from *the Swedish Research Council for Health, Working Life and Welfare* (Forte) supported the work of Jenny Cisneros Örnberg and Robin Room on the project. The research centre Eclectica and Collegio Carlo Alberto (University of Torino) have offered office space in Torino for the first author, which has greatly facilitated and speeded up the writing process. The University of Connecticut's Health Net, Inc., Endowed Chair in Community Medicine and Public Health provided support for the participation of Professor Thomas Babor in this project.

The authors would like to thank several individuals who provided invaluable help at various times in the production of the book. First, we thank Sara Rolando and Alice Scavarda for their arduous work in searching the relevant research literature and checking the references, Cesare Crova for the graphics, and Anna Alanko who provided invaluable help with checking the references and editing the manuscript. Anita Borch helped us with a report on the unique Norwegian experiences in gambling regulation, and Sara Rolando and Alice Scavarda wrote a summary report for this study on Italy, the biggest European gambling market. Maija Majamäki organized the collaborative meetings of the authors. We also acknowledge Peter Adams and Gerhard Bühringer, who contributed valuable advice during the early stages of the project, and Per Binde, whose comments on the manuscript are appreciated.

Finally, the authors thank their institutional affiliates for the time and resources provided to support work on this project.

Contents

Authors

Pekka Sulkunen, PhD, Professor Emeritus and former Director, Centre for Research on Addiction, Control and Governance (CEACG), Faculty of Social Sciences, University of Helsinki, Finland

Thomas F. Babor, PhD, MPH, Professor and Chairman, Department of Community Medicine, University of Connecticut School of Medicine Connecticut, United States of America

Jenny Cisneros Örnberg, PhD, Deputy Head of Department, Department of Public Health Sciences; Director, Centre for Social Research on Alcohol and Drugs (SoRAD), Stockholm University, Sweden

Michael Egerer, PhD, Researcher, Centre for Research on Addiction, Control and Governance (CEACG), Faculty of Social Sciences, University of Helsinki, Finland

Matilda Hellman, PhD, Research Director, Centre for Research on Addiction, Control and Governance (CEACG), Faculty of Social Sciences, University of Helsinki, Finland

Charles Livingstone, PhD, Senior Lecturer, School of Public Health and Preventive Medicine, Monash University, Melbourne, Australia

Virve Marionneau, PhD, Researcher, Centre for Research on Addiction, Control and Governance (CEACG), Faculty of Social Sciences, University of Helsinki, Finland

Janne Nikkinen, PhD, Docent in Social Ethics, University Researcher, Centre for Research on Addiction, Control and Governance (CEACG), Faculty of Social Sciences, University of Helsinki, Finland

Jim Orford, PhD, Professor Emeritus of Clinical and Community Psychology, University of Birmingham, United Kingdom

Robin Room, PhD, Professor, Department of Public Health Sciences and Centre for Social Research on Alcohol and Drugs (SoRAD); Professor, Centre for Alcohol Policy Research, La Trobe University, Melbourne, Australia

Ingeborg Rossow, PhD, Senior Researcher, Norwegian Institute of Public Health, Oslo, Norway

Chapter 1

Introduction

The complex nature of gambling problems

Commercial gambling has been progressively legalized since the mid twentieth century, and operates today as an industry in much of the world. This is an enormous change from what would have been true at the end of the Second World War. In the past, negative views on gambling so dominated the political agenda that it was often prohibited, sometimes with limited exceptions such as raffles, bets, and lotteries organized by churches, sports clubs, charities, and civil associations to cover their costs and to collect money for good purposes on a limited scale. Prohibition is still the official policy in large parts of the world, including most Islamic countries, but this situation is changing rapidly.

Gambling—placing a wager on a fortuitous event with a chance of winning it back with multiple value but also with a higher chance of losing it—is now being increasingly permitted by governments. The provision of gambling opportunities has become an industry of significant size, and the economic stakes have grown. At the same time governments have taken an interest in gambling as a source of revenue and other possible economic benefits. The legalization of gambling has often gone unnoticed and accepted as part of the tradition of earmarking some of the gambling proceeds to fund charitable, social, cultural, and sports activities (Kingma 2004). This has developed into an extensive web of dependencies between gamblers, game providers, public authorities, and the beneficiaries—associations and other institutions that deliver services and support for good causes on the basis of money coming from gamblers. On the other hand, as legalized gambling has expanded, there have been increases in social and psychological harms deriving from the activity. The adverse effects occur not only to gamblers, but also often to others in the family, the workplace, and the community. The issue of weighing benefits against harm is therefore complex. What is a benefit for one, or a source of 'voluntary tax' for a government, may cause serious harm to other parties, especially the players who run a risk of becoming obsessed about the game and ruining not only their own life chances but also those of others through excessive loss of money and property.

The need for more effective regulation is increasingly recognized, with the aim to limit and, where possible, prevent harms from gambling, and thus to serve the public good. The question is what forms of regulation serve this aim best. Policymakers must weigh policy options taking into account economic considerations, and consumers' freedom, as well as human suffering. Whatever the value priorities, inevitably the question will arise: what are the ways in which gambling markets can be organized and controlled? Drawing on the rapidly accumulating research on gambling practices and problems, and on regulatory measures and their effects, this book focuses on the answers that can be provided from the scientific study of gambling and gambling policies. Our aim is to inform policymakers and other stakeholders about the gravity of the problem, the issues to be resolved, and the effectiveness and consequences of different policy options. We recognize the complexity of gambling as a behavior and as an industry, with many forms and types of play, but also with a byzantine web of interests that connect policy consequences with business outcomes, the public economy, and a wide array of social activities funded from this source.

We are primarily concerned with gambling as an organized commercial activity carried on under governmental sanction and often supervision, with games of chance or bets as the main forms of the activity. In the 1950s a book on gambling policy would probably have focused on sports betting and games of skill like poker, played in clandestine settings, and the problems primarily addressed would have been fraud and crime. Today many previously criminal forms of gambling are legalized. Computerized games of pure chance attract the largest turnover in the majority of countries, and most of the activity is regulated by governments one way or another. Illegal gambling and gambling-related crime are still important issues, but most of the problems from the activity arise within the legal domain that governments can, will, and do regulate. This is why gambling policy today is a public issue with multiple dimensions that involves many different problems, professions, institutions, and government departments or ministries.

The first and most obvious gambling problem arises from excessive spending of money, which affects the individual, families, and other persons in the gambler's social environment. Financial issues are dealt with in financial counselling, social services, and the court system, and in Gamblers Anonymous, which has "pressure relief group meetings" where seasoned members help new members to deal with the immediate financial problems facing them.

The gambler's behavior is a second type of problem because it often damages intimate and family relationships by undermining trust, for instance by hiding the fact that resources which were owned in common have been bet and lost.

Relationship problems are commonly dealt with by psychologists, social workers, or marriage and family counselling agencies.

A third arena of gambling problems is crime. Gambling can be the cause of criminal activity, ranging from crime committed by problem gamblers in order to obtain funds, street crime around gambling establishments, or crimes violating gambling regulations, including organized criminality. Legal problems are typically dealt with by the criminal justice system.

Fourth, there are often health problems related to heavy gambling. They are dealt with by health care professions and institutions.

Problems related to gambling do not fit neatly under any one of these social rubrics. They can aggravate existing social problems, including socio-economic inequality and social alienation. Not only problem gambling, but also the activity in general can cause significant social costs. These types of problems are not easily dealt with by individual authorities.

The benefits from gambling are widely dispersed among businesses, beneficiary associations and local, national, and federal governments. The regulatory situation is exacerbated by the fact that the beneficiaries of gambling do not fall under the same purview as the related problems. The industry itself has an interest in avoiding problems that undermine their image and business success, and for this reason companies have developed "responsible gambling" strategies and codes of conduct.

The public interest approach to gambling

This book takes a public interest approach to gambling. This means that we discuss gambling issues from the perspective of what policies will best serve the public good, and minimize the individual and collective harms related to the activity. The approach is modelled on the public health approach, defined as what societies do collectively to advance the public good by assuring the conditions in which people can be healthy (Institute of Medicine 1988). While recognizing that gambling issues involve other dimensions along with health, we borrow from the public health paradigm the emphasis on the population as a whole rather than problem-behaving individuals. Furthermore, like the public health approach, we focus on inequalities within and between populations, accounting for structural and cultural dimensions in the occurrence of problems, as well as individual and interactional levels. Finally, in parallel with the public health approach, we do not take a stand on the moral worth of the activity itself. The public interest approach aims to promote the health and well-being of the public in terms of the consequences of gambling activities, stressing the role of government in advancing this goal.

This definition establishes a broad agenda for gambling policy. A narrower scope would only extend to prevention of problem gambling and treatment of gambling disorders. A common response has been to define gambling problems in terms of addiction and to manage them in ways similar to alcohol and drug problems. This choice confines the problem to defects in the individual gambler, rather than acknowledging that policy shifts and the expanding market are part of the problem. Depending on what theoretical background is used to frame the concept of addiction, some forms of gambling behavior may meet the criteria of this condition. A social science perspective relevant for prevention defines addiction as a loss of meanings, norms, and functions that normally regulate the behavior (Sulkunen 2015). A few studies have observed that one part of problem gambling behavior conforms to this definition (Sulkunen and Rantala 2012; Borch 2012). Nevertheless, confining the management of gambling within addiction services does not address the nature of the problems in the other arenas already described.

Our view contends that the problems of obsessively gambling individuals, however defined, are only a small part of the issue. Even within a public health agenda, broadly conceived, issues of inequality are essential. In gambling policy they are incontestable, and perhaps even more severe. Preventing problem behavior is in society's enlightened self-interest because it saves both money and suffering. We argue that a fair gambling policy must go even beyond that. Calculating costs and benefits to society is not a sufficient guide to a just and sound policy in this area, given that a large part of the benefits come from people who themselves need help, and go to people who can afford to meet their welfare needs without these contributions. Public interest in this case cannot be summed up as the balance of money spent and money earned, because the spenders and earners are not the same people.

What science offers the policymaker

Policymakers have had few opportunities to learn about gambling problems from a public interest perspective. The scientific study of gambling has improved substantially only in the past decade. For example, since 2000, more than 6,000 scientific articles have been published in the international literature, with more than half of them since 2010 (Babor et al. 2017). Much of this output has come from the United States (over 1,000 articles) with Canada, the United Kingdom, and Australia accounting for about the same amount of research collectively. A considerable amount of additional policy-relevant information and analysis comes from expert committee reports, investigative journalism, and other sources.

The types of research that can be applied to an understanding of gambling-related problems and to effective policy responses include experimental studies, quasi-experimental studies, survey research, and analyses of crime statistics. These types of research can inform us about the risk factors of problem gambling behavior. Some of them are related to individuals, others describe game features and gambling environments. Another set of studies focus on how gamblers spend their time and money, and on the harms resulting from gambling. A third type of research assesses the effects of gambling regulation not only on individuals but also on communities and society at large. Finally, treatment studies, especially clinical trials, inform us about the impact of interventions aimed at improving gamblers' own control of their behavior.

A major difficulty in gambling research is the complexity of causal attribution. As will become apparent in the following chapters, gambling is closely associated with mental disorders and addiction problems as well as poverty, but it is in most cases difficult to determine the causal path because these conditions often lead to and follow from excessive gambling behavior. This is an issue we shall address in the appropriate contexts of the analysis.

Another problem with gambling research is the potential for bias introduced by the influence of the gambling industry. A significant proportion of gambling research is funded by the industry itself or by organizations that serve as a conduit for industry research funds. For example, in the United States, a consortium of casinos and related companies set up the National Center for Responsible Gaming, which in turn funds other organizations that support research projects. As demonstrated in other areas of scientific research (Adams 2016; Babor and Miller 2014), industry funding can distort the research agenda, focusing it on topics which might help or at least are not likely to threaten industry interests. There is little evidence of bias in conclusions of the gambling research that has been conducted, but the research agenda is disproportionately focused on treatment rather than policy or prevention (Livingstone and Adams 2016). The proportion of research funded by the industry is impossible to estimate because many researchers do not declare their funding sources or conflicts of interest (Babor and Miller 2014). Nevertheless, several authorities on gambling and behavioral addictions (Schüll 2012; Adams 2016; Livingstone and Adams 2016) have raised concerns about the potential for bias created by industry support for research.

The moral dimensions and political economy of gambling

Gambling has long been under a moral cloud in many societies. Many religions condone at least some forms of gambling but others are more intolerant. Communist governments have often outlawed it. These days, affluent societies generally permit some access to gambling for adults, but even now public attitudes to gambling reflect considerable unease (Orford 2010).

In the present book, we seek to recognize this moral dimension but stand aside from judgments on the moral worth or censure regarding gambling itself as an activity. Rather it is one factor to enter in the assessment of its consequences and the effectiveness of gambling policy. A public interest framing involves built-in choices that can be regarded as having a moral dimension, just as other perspectives, such as consumers' rights or free market competition, have moral dimensions in privileging particular rights as principles to follow in government regulation. The aspects privileged in our analysis are the collective good and the minimization of harm, whether at the individual, interpersonal or collective levels.

This perspective leads us to include in the analysis not only the game and the gambler but also the political economy of gambling. Since the 1980s, the volume of gambling activities has increased substantially in the world. Modern consumer societies in the west and in many other parts of the world are characterized by greater moral diversity and less tolerance for restrictions on individual behavior than was the case even in the most industrially advanced countries until late in the twentieth century. As a consequence, gambling regulations have been relaxed and the public's access to gambling opportunities has increased. Crime prevention, and recently, more concern over tax evasion, fraud, and consumer safety in unregulated online gambling, have been used to justify the increased offer of legal and regulated gambling, both land-based and online.

Gambling is one of the economic fields in which operators produce a surplus far beyond the costs of providing the games, along with normal taxes like VAT or sales tax, and normal profits. This surplus, sometimes called 'rent' in economics and political science, is generated by many kinds of market imperfections, such as monopolistic pricing, consumer ignorance, patents and other forms of intellectual rights. In the case of gambling, even addiction may increase demand to an extent that defies normal balancing of supply and demand. Besides attractive returns for commercial investments, such a surplus provides a seemingly reliable and growing resource to fund welfare programs and other public expenses. In the European Union, gambling produces a public revenue of 85 billion EUR, which represents about 1.3% of the value of public spending. This share is similar in several other parts of the world, but in certain jurisdictions, such as the state of Nevada in the United States, this proportion can go up to 40%, and the economy and revenue in Macao, a small region in China, is almost entirely dependent on its casinos. In many countries this revenue is used to fund private or semi-private institutions that provide public services such as sports, culture, or health and social services, including associations and charities for the care of mental disorder, substance abuse, and other behavioral problems. In Finland about 60% of public subsidies provided to arts and cultural activities and 80% of support for sports emanate from revenue generated through gambling. For this reason, gambling has been aptly called a form of "voluntary taxation," applied especially since the onset of the neo-liberal turn in public sector management of western countries in the 1980s (Korn et al. 2003).

As will be explained in Chapter 3, governments' financial needs have proven to be a significant incentive to expand gambling in many countries. The growth in recent years of online gambling, often conducted across national boundaries, threatens the ability of governments to tax or otherwise harvest revenue from gambling, and thus presents a further inducement for them to protect national markets. This has been the case in Europe, where gambling provision has traditionally been under national state control, but also in the United States, where established land-based operators use lobbying at both state and federal levels to maintain their market positions. However, liberalizing regulations on gambling started in many countries *before* the internet became a relevant medium. Fiscal motives as well as ideological reasons probably explain the liberalizing trend better. It started contemporaneously with the deregulation of global financial markets, the rise of related neoliberal beliefs in consumer freedom, and pressure against taxes as the source of public funds. In several countries the gambling expansion has been justified as a non-tax-based way of funding public services and supporting state budgets.

Public policy and its vicious cycles

Public policy on gambling faces two problems, each one representing a sequence of reciprocal causes and effects. Figures 1.1 and 1.2 illustrate these as two types of vicious cycles. First, gambling produces public revenue which, simultaneously, generates costs due to gambling-related problems. This is what we call the First Loop. Secondly, vested interests in gambling revenue create a parallel Second Loop of financial dependency. Associations and other institutions that otherwise would be disposed to engage in prevention and to support preventive strategies are unable to act effectively because, if successful, this would reduce

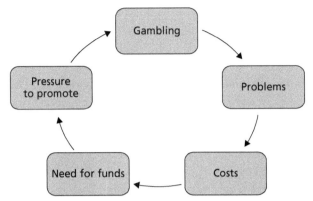

Fig 1.1 Cycle illustrating the First Loop—gambling generates public revenue to deal with costs due to gambling-related problems

their resources from gambling (Adams 2016). Support services for problem gamblers are funded in many countries directly by the public gambling companies. While it is fair that help is provided from resources generated by those who need it, the helping institutions may face a conflict of interest regarding efforts to reduce the gambling activities that they financially depend on.

Policymaking in practice is never just a matter of understanding causal connections between factors contributing to problems, and corresponding techniques to eliminate the causes. The feasibility of effective policy depends on institutional structures, the power of relevant interests, and modes of governance. The dependencies created by the money flows, or what we call the

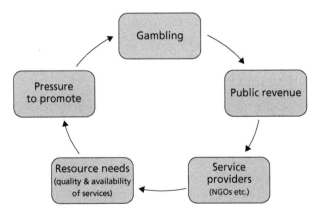

Fig 1.2 Cycle illustrating the Second Loop—gambling revenues are used to fund service providers who become financially dependent on the activity

Second Loop, complicate the policymaking process perhaps more than in other areas of public health, such as regulating alcohol or unhealthy food markets. Nevertheless, science does have a bearing on how policies perform in terms of their stated aims, and in raising issues which need to be considered in the public interest, such as protecting the consumer from aggressive marketing and the proliferation of gambling opportunities.

Objectives of this book

This book seeks to provide not only a thorough analysis of the vicious cycles of gambling problems, but also a window into concepts and scientific information that can be used to break the cycles. The central theme of this book is that when gambling problems are approached within the perspective of public interest, the opportunities for effective policies are enhanced dramatically. The ambition of this effort is to help policymakers, stakeholders, and nations to consider alternatives which might better serve the public interest, assist them in weighing the benefits and disadvantages of different policy approaches, and bring into these considerations an evaluated body of evidence.

The book has been written to answer the following fundamental questions about gambling policy:

- How can the historical background of gambling inform contemporary gambling policy at the local and national levels?
- What is the emerging global structure of the commercial gambling industry, and how does it compare with gambling activities managed by government monopolies and the informal sector?
- What is the prevalence of gambling behavior and gambling problems throughout the world, and how is it changing with the liberalization of gambling regulations?
- What are the personal, social and societal costs, and benefits of gambling, and do the costs outweigh the benefits?
- What can scientific research tell us about the policies and interventions that have been designed to regulate gambling, treat gambling disorders, and prevent gambling problems?

It will become clear from the answers provided to these questions that the combination of new gaming technologies, the concentration of gambling activities in large for-profit corporations, and the growth of state-sponsored gambling, have changed the cultural context and traditional roles of gambling at both the national and global levels. Any policy response motivated by the public interest will need to take these realities into account.

Chapter 2

The history of gambling regulation and the rise of the industry

From its ancient origins in small-scale gaming sites in local communities, gambling in the early twenty-first century has become a global industry and an increasingly standardized pastime across the world. The growth started in the early the 20th century, and accelerated in the past few decades. This expansion has not been straightforward. Gambling has been negatively viewed for religious, moral, and recently social reasons, which in most cases has led to extensive regulation by governments. Even today, parts of the world, most notably Islamic countries, continue to resist the spread of gambling (Orford 2010).

Gambling is not universal

The widespread diffusion of gambling practices across cultures has led some to postulate the existence of a 'gambling impulse', a universal desire to gamble that occurs in all societies and every period of history. Anthropologists Johan Huizinga (1938) and Roger Caillois (1958) are often quoted by proponents of this view, although their work refers to play in general and not to gambling specifically.

Other authors (Pryor 1976; Binde 2005) have identified specific factors that could account for variations in the amount of gambling in a society. According to Binde (2005), the presence of commercially used money, social inequality, societal complexity, and the practice of certain kinds of competitive inter-tribal rituals could explain the extent of gambling in a society.

Belief systems that associate desire for riches and social success with good luck have also been proposed to account for variations in gambling. Such beliefs contribute to fortune-seeking among the populations of many Eastern and South Asian countries, despite the disapproving influence of Buddhism, Islam, Hinduism, and Shintoism in the region (Warren 2013).

Regarding social structure, gambling has been nonexistent or strictly forbidden in nomadic societies and it is more likely to occur in fragmented societies. Pryor (1976) has shown that gambling is positively associated with socio-economic inequality, as it nurtures hope and dreams among the less fortunate.

Gambling appears to be more common among cultures where risk-taking is considered a positive character trait. Binde (2005) suggests that gambling is likely to be more prevalent in societies and groups where individual risk-taking is considered to be a positive character trait. Furthermore, dull and predictable surroundings may encourage the search for excitement in leisure activities such as gambling (Binde 2005).

Origins of modern gambling

Although gambling is not present in all civilizations, games of chance were incorporated into the cultural habits of some societies at a very early stage. In their early forms they were parts of religious rituals. The oldest known game of chance was to tell the mind of the divine with astragal bones or similar small objects in Mediterranean Europe, India, and Africa over ten thousand years ago (Schwartz 2006; David 1962; Thompson 2010). Many early religions have used similar instruments, such as the two-sided stones cast by Hebrew leaders to choose between alternative decisions (Thompson 2010), and colored stones commonly thrown by early Native Americans for divine guidance (Grant 1994). The function of these practices was to master uncertainty (Brenner and Brenner 1990). Similar practices are still common in Asian cultures today.

The advent of agriculture led to the creation of cities, the development of commerce, and the invention of money. This increased gambling dramatically in Mesopotamia, Babylonia, ancient Greece, Egypt, and Rome as well as in early Etruscan, Chinese, South American, and Egyptian civilizations (Schwartz 2006; Grant 1994). Box 2.1 provides a brief history of gambling in China, a country that exemplifies both its ancient roots and modern manifestations.

The roots of European gambling originate in the ancient cultures of the Middle East and Greece. The first records of horse racing date back to 4,000 BC in Babylonia, where soldiers used chariots in staged races. It is very likely that bets were wagered on them. Romans were eager bettors, and racing became an essential part of entertainment in the city state (Grant 1994). Merchants in the middle ages used the drawing of lots to dispose of items they were not able to sell otherwise (Thompson 2010). Lotteries became a common means of collecting public funds across Europe in the 15th and 16th centuries (Descotils and Guilbert 1993). The Catholic Church soon realized the potential of lotteries to fund the repair and building of churches (Neurisse 1991).

Casinos have their origins in Italy. The word comes from the Italian casa (home, house), designating aristocratic homes dedicated to entertainment. The first gambling houses started appearing in medieval Venice. Since the

Box 2.1 The evolution of gambling in China

China has probably the longest continuous history of gambling as an institution. By the Zhou dynasty (770–476 BC), gambling had already become a popular pastime in China as new games were gradually introduced. The first Chinese state lottery was thought to have been organized under the Tang Dynasty (618–907 CE). Gambling was further commercialized during the Northern and Southern Song Dynasties (960–1279), and by the Ming Dynasty (1368–1644), gambling dens flourished in major cities. Buddhist monasteries conducted lotteries to generate revenue. Card games originated in China, from where they were imported to Europe (David 1962). Imperial officials under the Qing Dynasty (1644–1911) found gambling dens to be a good source of tax revenue. The lower classes played games of dice, dominoes, and fantan; the upper classes enjoyed mahjong and lotteries (Lam 2014).

Modern casinos started to develop in China during the early 20th century. Games of chance from Western Europe became popular in the colonial consulates of Shanghai, adding one more vice to a city notorious for its prostitutes and opium addicts (Lam 2014). The Communist People's Republic of China of 1949 outlawed most gambling, and Mao's Cultural Revolution (1966–1976) suppressed it completely, with the exception of mahjong, which soon became very popular (Lam 2014).

After the Maoist regime, the Chinese welfare lottery was re-legalized in 1987, and a sports lottery was introduced in 1989 (Lam 2014). Gambling had been authorized in the Portuguese colony of Macau, where the first modern casino opened in 1937, when the Portuguese governor saw the potential to attract wealthy Chinese and European gentlemen to gamble. The development of gambling casinos continued after the Second World War, and Macau became officially a "tourism and gaming region" (Schwartz 2006). Today, Macau is the only place in China where casino gambling is legal, and by the late 20th century it had grown into one of the largest casino-gambling markets in the world.

12th century, authorities have attempted to keep gambling out of public sight, making gamblers relocate to small houses, *casini*. The first known casini date back to 1282 (Neurisse 1991).

In 17th-century Europe, and particularly in France, gambling became associated with luxury and excess. Most casino games popular today, including roulette, baccarat, and blackjack, were introduced around that time (Schwartz 2006), whereas poker in its various forms is a later American invention (Grant 1994).

The bourgeoisie disapproved of the conspicuous consumption of the nobility and started to distinguish between games of learning, suitable for the recreation of workers, and gambling, which was connected with idleness and immorality (Reith 1999). Gambling among the lower classes was restricted, allowed only during carnivals and other exceptional days of feasting. Between the 13th and 16th centuries, gambling prohibitions were lifted at Christmas time in many countries.

Until the 16th century, gambling had mainly been a matter of private bets and zero-sum games between individuals, but industrialization and urbanization of Europe during the 19th century turned gambling into commercial recreation. As modern tourism developed, casinos were opened in the Rhine valley, Baden-Baden, and Wiesbaden in Germany, Normandy in France, and other leisure destinations. Swiss casinos became fashionable, and counted famous personalities such as Dostoyevsky among their customers (Neurisse 1991). The French Riviera became the main gambling destination of Europe and the world. Monaco developed into the European model of casino tourism in this period (Schwartz 2006). Casinos were placed away from major urban centers, mainly to protect the working classes and the local bourgeoisie (Parvulesco 2008). Public houses were places where innkeepers provided gamblers with cards and dice, and also lent money. Gambling and drinking formed natural bedfellows and became to many a symbol for social decay (Kavanagh 2005).

Some native populations in India, Oceania, and North America had established gambling practices already before colonization (Binde 2007a). Native American tribes of every linguistic group had dice games. Clifford Geertz's (2011) famous account of Balinese cock-fighting has demonstrated that gambling had a high symbolic value among some indigenous populations in South-East Asia. Other native populations in the Pacific region, Western Australia, and New Zealand had no known gambling practices prior to colonialist settlement (Schwartz 2006; Breen 2008).

The European colonial expansion spread European games to many parts of the world. The British East India Company introduced horse racing and card games into South Asia in the mid-18th century. Gambling was imported into Australia and New Zealand by the new, mainly British, settlers. Early arrivers were mostly soldiers, sailors and convicts, groups who were familiar with gambling and brought their habits with them (Breen 2008; Grant 1994). Upper class English settlers continued to bet at race tracks and played card games, euchre, and vingt-et-un.

British and Spanish settlers introduced lotteries to their colonies (Thompson 2010). By the mid-18th century, colonial lotteries had become an important source of funds for building bridges and roads and to finance universities, churches, and libraries in all of the original 13 colonies in North America (Dunstan 1997; Neurisse 1991).

The popularity of gambling in the United States further increased in the 19th century. New Orleans was the original gambling capital of the country. The first casino was opened there in 1828. Following the Civil War, the state legislature also authorized the infamous Louisiana Lottery that sold tickets across the United States, defying a general ban on lotteries. From New Orleans, casino gambling spread inland on the riverboats of the Mississippi and Ohio River. After the Civil War in 1865, gambling spread to the west along railroad lines.

The end of the 19th century also saw the introduction of coin-in-the-slot machines, or slot machines. The first of these, the Liberty Bell, was introduced in San Francisco in 1895 (Schwartz 2006). Its three reel design is still used in some slot machines today. Entertainment machines originally demanding dexterity to win, the "Bajazzo", were popular in Europe in the early 20th century (Meyer and Bachmann 2011). Electronic gambling machines (EGMs) started to develop in the second half of the 20th century, first simulating slot machines and games of skill, and later incorporating computerized information technologies. They now involve no element of skill (Woolley and Livingstone 2010). An important innovation by the American EGM developer Bally's was the introduction of progressive machines, which permitted jackpots to grow each time a player made a losing play (Thompson 2010).

The alcohol prohibition years (1919–1933) in the United States, which eliminated legal drinking places as locales for commercial gambling, saw a general rise of gambling industries outside the United States but near the border. Caribbean and South American casinos tempted American players with luxurious casino hotels.

The expansion of the gambling industry

The expansion of the gambling industry continued in the non-communist world in the 20th century with democratization of the practice, as casinos and horse races were made accessible to the middle and working classes.

Two waves of expansion can be distinguished, the first between or in some cases after the two World Wars and the second since the 1980s. The need to reconstruct Europe after the First World War gave birth to gambling monopolies that would collect public funds (Turay 2007). In France, for instance, a lottery by the name of La Dette (the debt) was introduced in 1931 to collect funds for disabled veterans of the First World War, and was soon institutionalized as the National Lottery.

The stock market crash in 1929 and the ensuing depression were used to justify gambling in the United States. Nevada began to relax its gambling laws in the 1930s. The city of Reno became an important gambling destination with casinos, bingo parlors, and slot machines. Soon after, the Las Vegas gambling industry was born. "The Strip" started developing in the 1940s (Thompson 2010). The post-war prosperity and democratization of gambling practices brought along the transition from small scale gambling halls to glittering mass gambling resorts, as Las Vegas became a holiday destination for average Americans (Schwartz 2006).

Commercial gambling continued its gradual growth until a second wave of expansion began in the 1980s. The most important developments have been the concentration of casinos in Macao and Atlantic City, the establishment of commercial gambling on Native American tribal reservations in the United States and First Nations reserves in Canada, and the growth of gambling machines in community clubs in Australia (Thompson 2010). The US gambling industry grew tenfold between 1976 and 1998, with casinos and racinos (horse racing tracks that also offer casino games) making most of the profit (Orford 2010).

An important driver of growth-promoting policy in Europe as elsewhere has been the desire to keep gambling revenues within the local jurisdiction. For example, the population in Finland participated widely in Swedish lotteries before the introduction of the Finnish National Lottery in 1940 (Matilainen 2010). A similar process can be seen in the United States: the introduction of lotteries in the early 1970s, scratch tickets in the late 1970s, and casinos since the 1980s. When one state introduces a game that is not available elsewhere, neighboring states usually follow (Thompson 2010).

The first gambling websites started to appear in 1995 and 1996, increasing the speed of expansion of the gambling market around the globe. Many countries declared internet gambling illegal to protect their own gambling schemes against operators registered in more tolerant jurisdictions. The small Caribbean nation of Antigua, as well as Gibraltar and Malta in Europe, have become known for their massive offshore gambling operations.

Restrictions and regulations

The story of gambling includes a rich history of oscillation between restriction and permissiveness (Rose 1991). How societies regard it has vacillated between prohibition motivated by moral or religious concerns and active promotion motivated by profit-seeking and state financial needs. Restrictive efforts have occurred in different historical contexts, depending on what kind of danger or harm the activity is seen as representing.

Monotheistic world religions tend to condemn gambling as an impious belief in forces that defy God's will (Binde 2007a). The Quran condemns gambling as a violation of Allah's authority to promote the prosperity of the faithful, and consequently countries with Islamic governments have outlawed it for 1,500 years. Prohibitions by Islamic law are rigorously enforced in Saudi Arabia, Iran, and Pakistan, where the government filters access to international gambling websites. The Turkish Islamic government has not been able to eliminate all gambling in the country and on the internet, despite a prohibition that took effect in 1998. The illegal and irreligious status of gambling in Islamic countries is not the only reason why gambling has failed to develop. In Islamic countries, gambling never assumed the image of a pastime of the rich and powerful, as it did in North America and non-Islamic countries in Asia and Europe (Rosenthal 1975).

Unlike the Quran, the Bible does not condemn gambling. Christians' views depend on the denomination. The Catholic Church and the Church of England have banned gambling by the clergy and have regarded some games like dice negatively, associating them with pagan origins. However, the lottery has been accepted since the 18th century and has even been organized by churches (Neurisse 1991). Both denominations accept gambling today, but are critical of its contemporary commercial forms (Egerer et al. 2016). The Lutheran Protestant churches in Northern Europe are also more accepting of state-organized gambling.

The first wave of strong anti-gambling sentiment in modern Europe followed the Protestant Reformation in the 16th and 17th centuries. Protestant Pietism considered time to be as valuable as money. Gambling was seen to waste both, to destroy families and encourage idleness, greed, blasphemy, and superstition. Christian groups with Puritan heritage such as Methodists still condemn gambling in all circumstances as the work of the devil and as a sin, which stands in opposition to the values of hard work and austerity, as do Protestant-derived sects such as the Latter-Day Saints (Mormons) (Reith 2006).

As concern over industrial workers emerged in the 19th century, industrialization placed gambling in the framework of the "social question". It was considered a threat to the working class and disruptive for the social order. For example, legislation in Britain raised minimum stakes in lotteries to keep them out of reach of the poor. In North America, legislation was drafted to prevent the lower social classes from participating. In line with these traditions, but also reflecting collectivist values, communist countries in the Soviet era, and contemporary China, officially banned gambling. Box 2.2 illustrates the political

Box 2.2 Gambling in Russia and the Soviet Union

Gambling was very popular in tsarist Russia, with casino games, lotteries, and racetracks tempting both upper and lower class players, despite legal ambiguity. Card games were prohibited from the middle of the 17th century onwards until Catherine the Great made the distinction between authorized 'games of commerce' and illegal 'games of chance'. Despite its illegal status, gambling was nevertheless popular among the aristocracy (Tsytsarev and Gilinsky 2009). The Gambler, a novel by Fyodor Dostoyevsky, and The Queen of Spades, an opera by Pyotr Tchaikovsky, are widely-known artistic presentations of the propensity to gamble that has been described as a peculiarity of the Russian people (Shepel 2007).

The founding of the Soviet Union in 1917 changed the situation dramatically. The Bolsheviks considered gambling as a corrupt bourgeois activity that had no place in the new communist society. Gambling houses were closed down in areas populated by workers, and in 1928 all gambling establishments across the Soviet territory were officially banned. Only state and local lotteries as well as bets at horse races were exempt from the ban (Tarasov 2010). The first horse races were organized in 1921 and they became popular among wealthy bettors and those who wanted to launder their illegal income (Tsytsarev 2008).

A new lottery Sportloto was introduced in 1976 to fund the Moscow Olympics in 1980. In 1988, 226 slot machines were installed in Intourist hotels to cater to foreign visitors in Moscow, Leningrad, Sochi, and Yalta. The first Soviet casino opened its doors in Tallinn, Estonia, in 1989. There is no statistical data on gambling in the Soviet Union, but according to Tsytsarev (2008), the practice was very widespread, and lottery participation was encouraged by the Soviet government.

vicissitudes of lotteries and gambling in Russia and the Soviet Union since the days of the tsars.

The European moral environment of the 19th century was strict concerning the leisure activities, sexuality, and alcohol consumption of the lower classes. Those attitudes also extended to gambling. The last British lottery was held in 1826, to be restarted only a century later. A general ban on all gambling was introduced in France in 1836. The European anti-gambling sentiment continued up to the First World War (Orford 2010). The alcohol Prohibition movement at the turn of the 20th century also brought bans on gambling in the

United States. The last casinos were closed in 1910. The gambling ban lasted until 1931, when casinos were again legalized, starting in Nevada.

There was general uncertainty regarding the legality of gambling in Canada until 1892, when the Canadian Parliament banned most forms of gambling. Only horse racing and games at fairs were legal until amendments were made to the Criminal Code in 1969 and 1985.

The Australian colonial administration was initially permissive, but gambling in Asian groups who came to the goldfields or as laborers was prohibited (Australian Productivity Commission 1999). Private gambling clubs were accessible only to the European immigrants, but they started to receive negative attention after the Second World War. The New South Wales (NSW) Gaming and Betting Act of 1956 gave registered clubs in NSW the exclusive right to operate gambling machines. Since the 1980s, gambling opportunities have again been increasingly privatized and gambling machines have become more broadly available in other states (Australian Productivity Commission 1999).

During the 20th century, the status of European gambling changed. National lotteries were set up in many European countries after the First World War. Income taxes were still a minor and insufficient source to fund war reconstruction, veteran care, and mounting costs of public services in social, health, and cultural areas. In line with public revenue from excise duties and other fees on many commodities, gambling became an attractive source to finance public services, whether directly through government ministries or through revenue to be used by NGOs for "good causes". The emphasis in gambling policies shifted from moral control to satisfying state and charitable financial needs. The aim was also to stop an influx of foreign lottery tickets that imported potential problems but exported financial benefits. Lotteries and national betting monopolies became symbolic institutions of national solidarity, due to the good causes they supported (Matilainen 2010).

Market orientation

The 1980s saw a new orientation in gambling policy worldwide. Deregulation of the financial markets, combined with digitalization, started a new era of globalized capital flows, and this also affected gambling markets. In a neoliberal era giving primacy to market freedoms, restrictions were removed to allow development of gambling industries as a valued element of the national economy. With this orientation, a permissive approach no longer has to be justified by what Kingma (2004) calls the *alibi* model, i.e., fiscal concerns or interest in funding good causes. Rather, the economic activity generated by the gambling industry itself has come to be seen as positive. Orford (2010) suggests that there was such a change in public discourse in the United Kingdom between the

1968 and 2005 Gambling Acts. Initially, the rhetoric focused on meeting un-stimulated demand for gambling. This was replaced by a free market rationale and governmental encouragement of gambling. In Australia, the Australian Productivity Commission (1999) noted a change of rationale from social con-siderations to economic opportunities. Similar trends have been described in the Netherlands (Kingma 2004).

Such changes have occurred even in countries that have resisted gambling. Tourism has been an important incentive to introduce gambling despite reli-gious concerns. In Malaysia, for example, casino gambling is allowed for tour-ists and non-Muslim locals. A Muslim religious organization is allowed to patrol the casino and to eject and punish any local Muslim it finds (Thompson 2010).

The new government in South Africa introduced a competitive casino in-dustry after the end of the apartheid regime, legitimizing this move in terms of expected economic benefits for indigenous peoples (Sallaz 2010). In the Philippines, several governmentally operated casinos have become popular. The country had not been subject to the religious restraints of most Asian coun-tries, since it had been under Spanish and US control until 1946 with strong, gambling-tolerant Catholic influences (Thompson 2010).

Today, governments are facing unprecedented international competition. Investors seeking growth potential have been interested in new markets for gambling products, but also pressure from gambling across state borders has influenced the way governments rethink their gambling policies.

However, pressures for a single market in Europe have had the paradoxical effect of pushing member states towards more restrictive rather than more lib-eral gambling policies (Kingma 2008). The paradox arises from efforts by some national governments to protect the revenues of national gambling monop-olies from the cross-border free trade rules of the European Union. The Court of Justice of the European Union has insisted that justifications of such monop-olies on public health or public interest grounds require a good-faith effort to be acting in the interest of public health (Room and Cisneros Örnberg 2014). Restrictive measures such as age limits, marketing regulations, and identity controls at casinos have been introduced in many European Union member states, not only to protect consumers but also as part of the good-faith effort.

In the 21st century, there have been new efforts in a number of jurisdictions to rein in gambling by controlling availability. Norway limited EGM gambling drastically in 2006, South Carolina in the United States removed EGMs com-pletely, and Russia confined all gambling to four gambling zones at the outer limits of the country in 2009. These examples reflect a new concern about gam-bling as a social issue.

The rise of problem gambling as a policy target

The 19th century concern about gambling considered it to be a social problem rather than an individual pathology. As gambling has become a form of mass entertainment, and as the economic stakes have grown for the industry, for governments, and for the "good causes" funded under the alibi model, the moral and disciplinary walls around gambling have eroded. "Problem gambling" was distinguished from other gambling, and the gambling issue was redefined from the temptations of a questionable activity to the behavior of problematic individuals who were unable to control their impulses. The worry about some people spending more than they can afford, hurting themselves and others, and possibly becoming addicted, is a major consideration in gambling policy even in countries with an industry of substantial size, and within a policy that is otherwise favorable towards it. This means that the problem has become individualized, and in some measure even medicalized.

The first efforts in this direction came with psychoanalysis in the early 20th century. Sigmund Freud, the founder of psychoanalysis, identified gambling as an addiction (Ferentzy and Turner 2013). Another disease model was later adopted by the Gamblers Anonymous movement that was established in Los Angeles in 1957. The movement was influenced by Alcoholics Anonymous, and problem gambling was modelled after its concepts (Rosecrance 1985). Another development of the mid-20th century was the application of learning theory, particularly operant conditioning models, to different forms of gambling, and especially to gambling on EGMs. The theory was particularly important in explaining why even ordinary people, and not only those with underlying mental health issues, could become problem gamblers. The insights of operant conditioning have been developed into cognitive and behavioral therapies to help individuals with gambling problems (Ferentzy and Turner 2013).

Further medical approaches to identify individuals with elevated risk, and to help those who have difficulty in controlling their participation, have been influenced by advanced knowledge of brain functioning, and this has precipitated the search for effective pharmacological treatments.

The medical approach has been particularly popular in the United States. On the other hand, many European and Australian researchers (e.g., Livingstone and Woolley 2007) have criticized the medical models, instead framing problem gambling as a social issue. In Australia, Canada, and Northern Europe, a wider public health model has emerged (e.g., Adams, Raeburn and de Silva 2009; Korn and Shaffer 1999). In China, problem gamblers have been considered undesirable to society rather than sick (Lam 2014).

Conclusion: history and the future of gambling

Wherever and whenever gambling has existed, those in political power have sought to control it, and this remains true in both democratic and non-democratic countries. Islamic and communist regimes have been most consistently negative for moral reasons. There have also been periods of prohibition or stringent restriction in countries dominated by the Protestant Christian faith, reflecting values that rewards should be honestly earned through work, rather than by chance. Controls on gambling became part of the "social question" after the industrial revolution, with controls and even prohibition targeting the working classes while the wealthy began to visit casinos in emerging tourist destinations in the 19th century. Total prohibitions at a national level were common until the end of the First World War, when governments turned to lotteries to finance their growing fiscal needs, which included the added expenses of the nascent 'welfare state' and the provision of support for war casualties. National lotteries and charity gambling became symbols of national solidarity, and grew further in size in the three decades after the Second World War. This period also saw commercial gambling starting to develop in the United States.

Policy concern about problem gambling as a harmful behavior and as a condition of the gambling individual re-emerged with the substantial growth in gambling provision, and became prominent in the context of the rise of the industry and of increased levels of gambling since the 1980s.

Despite the policy changes allowing a massive increase in gambling markets, even today gambling is seen negatively by the majority of the population in countries where their opinions have been surveyed. In the face of this opinion, governments must struggle to seek a balance between the societal benefits of the activity, the prevention of fraud and crime, and the harm caused by this industry. The following chapters will analyze in detail the issues involved in weighing the costs and benefits against each other, keeping in mind that the benefits and harms do not go to the same groups and individuals in competitive societies.

Chapter 3

The gambling industry: global structures and modern trends

By the late twentieth century, gambling markets had assumed global dimensions, and this trend has accelerated since then. It has become an industry intertwined with tourism, entertainment, professional sports and the media. This expansion has occurred in close connection with the commercialization of gambling, which has been facilitated by governments in the interest of generating employment, increasing public revenues, and supporting charities and associations that provide valuable public services. This chapter describes the growth of the gambling industry in terms of its volume, structure, and the distribution of different types of games in different parts of the world.

Global growth in gambling

Figure 3.1 shows the global growth in the volume of recorded gambling measured as the Gross Gambling Revenue (GGR). GGR is the sum of all money gambled minus the winnings returned to players. It can be considered as the sum of private net expenditures, or *losses* on gambling, and it thus describes the sum of money that consumers spend on gambling activities. The volume of gambling has grown at a steady rate and it is estimated to exceed 400 billion EUR in 2019. The growth has been greatest in North America, Asia, and the Middle Eastern region. Africa and Latin America have only seen a modest growth. By 2010 Asia had surpassed the United States as the largest market in the world. The decline in Asia in 2014–2015 is due to the Chinese government's anti-corruption policies. European national markets may be saturating, facing competition against online supply by international operators (Browne 2015; Bland 2015).

Average (per capita) gambling expenditures are calculated as GGR divided by the number of adult residents. It is usually not possible to calculate the amount of money tourists or people under the permissible age limit contribute to the total. As shown in Figure 3.2, losses per capita are highest in Australia with the exception of Singapore, but it should be noted that the latter country hosts a large amount of casino tourism from abroad. The United States is the world's largest gambling market with a GGR of 94 billion EUR; China including Macao

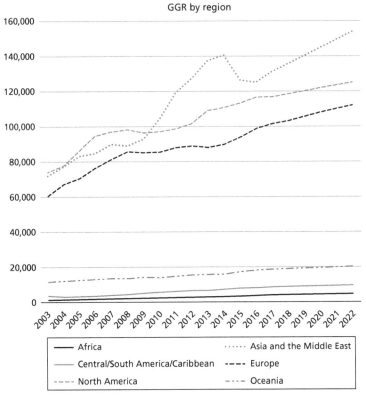

Fig 3.1 Annual Gross Gambling Revenue (GGR) in million EUR by global regions between 2003 and 2022. Figures for 2018–2022 are estimates.
Data courtesy of H2 Global Gambling Capital.

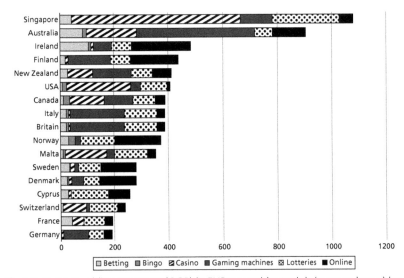

Fig 3.2 Gross Gambling Revenues (GGR) in EUR per resident adult (average losses) by type of game in 2017 in 17 countries.
Data courtesy of H2 Global Gambling Capital.

and Hong Kong (data not included in Figure 3.2) is second with its GGR of 50 billion EUR.

Expenditures on various games differ significantly among countries, co-varying with total spending (Figure 3.2). Countries with high overall gambling expenditures tend to spend proportionately larger amounts in casinos and on electronic gambling machines (EGMs) outside casinos. In Australia, the average gambling losses on casinos and EGMs outside casinos amounted to about 618 EUR per resident adult, more than half of the total. In Finland, a country ranking fourth on gambling losses per resident adult, losses in the casino and on EGMs were 169 EUR per adult in 2017. This was more than a third of the Finnish GGR total of 1.6 billion EUR. According to the H2 Gambling Capital data, casinos and EGMs outside casinos accounted for 30.7 billion EUR in gambling losses in the EU member states in 2012. This constituted 38% of all gambling losses in the area. Interactive gambling (on internet and mobile devices) accounted for 10.6 billion EUR in gambling losses in 2012, which was 13% of total gambling losses that year. Gambling losses increased by 54% in the European Union over a decade from 56 billion EUR in 2003 to 80 billion EUR in 2012.

Most of this increase can be attributed to the increase in spending on interactive games and slot machines. Gambling with computers actually has stopped growing after 2010. Instead access to gambling via mobile devices (telephones, tablets) is growing vigorously, as is shown in Figure 3.3.

Unrecorded and illegal gambling

A common problem in gambling research is that a large part of the activity captured is neither in the overall volume figures nor in gambling prevalence estimates. This undetected part is called *unrecorded gambling*. This and other terms important for an understanding of modern trends in gambling are defined in Box 3.1. Detecting and deterring unrecorded gambling is one of the main concerns of public gambling policy. Government control agencies and legal market operators are interested in unrecorded gambling not only because of the harms associated with an illicit market but also because of its competition with the legal market and the revenue loss it entails for the government and for licensed interests.

Illegal gambling satisfies demands that legitimate providers are unable to address, in part because it takes forms not allowed in the legitimate market. One example is poker, which is typically organized in private circles (Piedallu 2014) but also provided online, often by unauthorized companies.

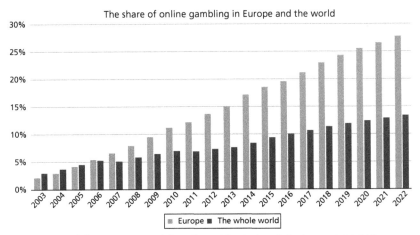

Fig 3.3 Growth in access to gambling via mobile devices (telephones, tablets) in Europe and the entire world. The upper figure displays the share of total gambling from mobile devices by year. The lower figure displays revenues? from gambling with mobile devices in millions of euros by yea. Figures for 2018–2022 are estimates.
Data courtesy of H2 Global Gambling Capital.

Another example is sports betting. It has been estimated that 80% of the global sports betting market is illegal, representing between 225 billion and 547 billion EUR (Sender 2014). In the United States, only Oregon and Nevada allow sports betting, leaving room for a vast underground sector. According to one estimate (Sherman 2017), Americans wagered approximately 121 billion EUR on illegal online gambling sites. In Germany, governmental officials estimate that the annual turnover of the unauthorized sports betting market is 2.7 billion EUR, of which about 60% is generated online (European Commission 2012).

Other cases of unauthorized gambling include clandestine EGMs and computer terminals that have been turned into gambling machines, common in bars in southern France, Greece, and Spain, and mafia-controlled gambling machines in Italian pubs (Spapens 2014; Trucy 2006). A number of illegal gambling houses began operating in Russia after the gambling reform of 2006 restricted the availability of legal gambling opportunities to four jurisdictions that were located in remote areas (Tsytsarev and Gilinsky 2009).

The proportion of gambling which is illegal may be even more significant outside Western countries. Nations that have maintained bans on gambling until recently often have large clandestine markets. The illegal Brazilian animal

Box 3.1 Definitions of key terms used in gambling on the margins of regulation

Unrecorded gambling: This includes illegal or unauthorized forms of gambling that take place outside the perimeters of officially licensed providers in a specific jurisdiction. It also includes legal gambling that is not identified by the tools to measure gambling activity.

Unregulated gambling: Gambling that is not authorized in the specific country, but authorized elsewhere. Many companies such as Betsson, Casino Cottage, Mr. Green, and PokerStars operate across borders in this way. It is not illegal to play games operated by such companies and legal authorities in most countries do not interfere with the business, which has the permission of the country where it is based. So it is neither permissible nor impermissible, legal nor illegal; it is unregulated.

Illegal gambling: Gambling that is prohibited by law. For example, an underground club open to the public where customers can play cards for money, or gambling machines that are placed in a pizzeria without a proper licence. Many countries attempt to outlaw online operators from outside their borders.

Unregistered gambling: This occurs when a person buys a gaming product anonymously. In Sweden, for example, this takes place when a person: a) buys a physical scratch card, b) plays at a restaurant casino, c) buys betting tickets over the counter in a shop or on the racetrack, d) buys lottery tickets in a store or from ambulatory vendors.

lottery, *Jogo de bicho,* has been estimated to collect almost 60% more revenue than legal lotteries (Medeiros et al. 2016a). In India, clandestine lottery sales account for about half the Indian gambling market (an estimated 48 billion EUR per year) (Benegal 2012).

As access to the internet has spread, online gambling has become a particular concern of both private gambling providers and national finance authorities in their attempt to restrict cross-border betting. Illegal and unregulated online gambling have grown dramatically in recent years. Data from the Canadian province Québec shows that 17% of online gambling took place via illegal channels in 2002, rising to 32% in 2009 (Leblond 2013). In many EU countries unregulated online gambling represents much higher proportions of the total. For example, the government of Slovakia estimates that 90% of online players gamble on mostly unauthorized foreign sites (European Commission 2012).

The role of policy in the growth of the gambling industry

The growth of unregulated and illegal online gambling has increased the borderless nature of the gambling market, but it does not account for the dramatic expansion of the global gambling industry. The global expansion of the gambling market was in fact under way before the growth of the internet became a relevant factor.

Gambling participation was increasing well before the introduction of the internet, as it was associated with govenments' efforts to legalize and regulate the activity. State lotteries were often the first forms of gambling offered to the general public, sometimes justified as an alternative to tax increases. Other changes that increased opportunities to gamble included the introduction of new casinos or the relaxation of restrictions on EGMs. Such liberalizations occurred in the United States (Thompson 2010), Canada (Korn 2000; Smith 2014), New Zealand (Adams 2004), Australia (especially Victoria) (Livingstone 2005), China (Lam 2014), South Africa (Sallaz 2010), the United Kingdom (Orford 2010), France (Bégin 2001), Italy (Rolando and Scavarda 2016), Norway (Borch 2012), Finland (Tammi 2008), the Netherlands (Kingma 2004), Poland (Dzik 2009), and Russia (Kassinove, Tsytsarev, and Davidson 1998). Amusement machines with prizes (AWPs), offering low stakes and payouts, initially involving an element of skill, were already available in Germany when the industry upgraded these to EGMs with significant stakes and jackpots during the 1980s. Circumvention of the German prohibition of EGMs outside casinos was challenged by legislators only in the mid-2000s. In all of these cases participation in, and spending on, gambling increased after the liberalizing reforms.

Deregulating one gambling sector tends to create a 'domino effect' in which other sectors then press for further deregulation (Adams 2004). For example, after a lottery regulation reform in Norway in 1986, charitable organizations lost the income they had obtained from small scale lotteries. As compensation, they were permitted to set up EGMs, which significantly increased the availability of these devices in Norway (Rossow and Hansen 2016). A similar process took place in France, where new games introduced by the National Lottery (*La Française des Jeux*) and National Pari-Mutuel betting company (PMU) saw the popularity of the casino industry decline in the 1980s. As a result, the legislature was persuaded to allow casinos to operate EGMs (Bégin 2001).

Through state lotteries, national monopolies, licence fees or tax revenues from casinos, national or state/provincial governments (or both levels) are closely linked to the gambling industry in many countries. This creates strong vested interests. Federal or national governments have stronger concerns for gambling-related harm than lower jurisdictional levels in countries where the regional jurisdictions have constitutional authority only for a limited range of conventional taxes but simultaneous responsibilities for social, health, and cultural services. The Canadian provinces have the exclusive right to manage gambling, which has resulted in the growth of casinos, EGMs, and gambling revenues across the country (Korn 2000). In Australia, gambling taxes in the federal state of Victoria made up 14.3% of its taxation by the year 2002, following the liberalization of gambling in 1991 (Livingstone 2005). The Indian Gaming Regulatory Act of 1988 in the United States was based on a similar rationale of opening up gambling as a source of revenue on reservations for tribal authorities. The federal act allows indigenous communities to open casinos and offer other forms of gambling on their tribal land, if the particular form is allowed anywhere else in the state in which the reservation is located, and to support community causes with the proceeds. The introduction of a competitive gambling market in South Africa following the end of apartheid was similarly justified in terms of benefiting indigenous groups (Sallaz 2010). In these circumstances, federal or national governments tend to have stronger concerns for gambling-related harm than lower jurisdictional levels.

On the other hand, in several European countries gambling returns support the national or federal budgets, whereas lower level jurisdictions bear the burden of related problems, making them favorable to preventive efforts (Egerer, Maironneau, and Nikkinen 2018).

The South African example demonstrates that changes in gambling legislation often follow wider and more encompassing political changes. Central and Eastern European countries and Russia experienced an abrupt change from a planned economy to a market economy after the dissolution of the Soviet Union in 1991. As general restrictions on private enterprise disappeared, many previously outlawed forms of gambling were permitted since there were no gambling-specific restrictive policies in place.

Box 3.2 provides a case study of the casinos of Macau, which illustrates the unique role played by government policy in the growth of the international gambling industry.

North America, Europe and Asia have been the front-runners of gambling expansion in terms of market size and volume among the continents. Asia, with 33% of the world market in 2015, is the largest gambling area, the position held by North America until 2010. In each of these regions, it has been the liberalization of government restrictions that has permitted the growth of the industry.

Box 3.2 The casino industry in Macau

The Chinese island of Macau, within one-hour's ferry ride of Hong Kong, occupies a prominent place in the global gambling market. The Portuguese colonial government legalized traditional Chinese games of chance in 1847. Monopoly privileges were given to two companies in the 1930s for baccarat and other games. In 1962, the monopoly in casino games was given to Sociedade de Turismo e Diversoes de Macao (STDM) for forty years.

Gambling was outlawed in mainland China when the communist regime took over in 1949. After Macau became part of China in 1999, exceptional rules allowing gambling were continued, monopoly rights were dissolved and the number of companies increased. Australian and Las Vegas casino interests entered the market.

In the decade before 2013, gambling revenues increased eightfold (Browne 2015). Besides international tourists, the main gambling revenue has come from affluent, high-stakes gamblers from mainland China. One estimate places the amount of illegal gambling in China at about 1.4 billion EUR, a significant amount in a country that supposedly does not have much gambling, but modest (about 10% of the Australian total) for a population of 1.3 billion (Eimer 2010).

A Chinese government campaign against corruption launched in 2013 reduced Macau gambling revenues dramatically. In 2015, the profits of the six largest casino operators in Macau dropped by 40% compared to 2014 (Browne 2015; Bland 2015). Chinese authorities want Macau to diversify its economy, currently generating at least 80% of its income from gambling-related activities. The Chinese government decided in 2017 to limit the right of managerial employees in public office to gamble in Macau, which has substantially cut down the operations of global gambling companies in the province.

EGMs as drivers of increased gambling revenues

Another way of describing the volume of gambling is to count the number of EGMs within a jurisdiction. This provides a rough estimate of availability of gambling. The top 10 countries with EGMs are shown in Table 3.1.

The exceptionally high Japanese figure is attributable to Pachinko machines that do not offer wins in money. Wins are provided in the form of toys and other articles that can be exchanged for money in special shops.

EGMs generate much, if not most of the profit for the gambling industry, and most of the harm caused by it. Casinos are supposedly designed to cater to 'high rollers' interested in table games, but in reality most of their profit is derived from EGMs. EGMs were banned in most Australian jurisdictions until the 1990s, and remain banned outside casinos in Western Australia, where GGR per capita is half that in the rest of Australia. Where they were available, the bets that could be placed were relatively small. "Pokies," or slot machines, were also very basic, and lacked modern features such as linked jackpots and the ability to bet on multiple lines simultaneously. There are now over 195,000 EGMs in Australia, with 98,000 in the state of New South Wales alone (The Economist 2017). EGMs today increasingly encourage betting in high amounts (Markham and Young 2014). Multi-line EGMs are very effective devices for maximizing

Table 3.1 Number of Electronic Gambling Machines (EGMs) in different countries and persons per machine in ten countries with the world's biggest EGM market in 2016

Jurisdiction/rank	Number of EGMs	Persons/machine
1. Japan	4,575,545	28
2. Australia	197,122	122
3. Italy	456,367	132
4. Spain	212,153	219
5. Germany	277,325	298
6. Canada	98,902	369
7. United States	865,807	373
8. United Kingdom	167,839	391
9. Argentina	98,717	444
10. Mexico	90,000	1,417

Data sourced from Ziolkowski S. The World Count of Gaming Machines (2016) the Gaming Technologies Association http://gamingta.com/wp-content/uploads/2016/10/World_Count_of_Gaming_Machines_2015.pdf.

gambling revenue. At the time of writing it is possible to place a bet of up to 100 GBP and lose it within 20 seconds in a fixed-odds betting terminal in a UK High Street betting shop, or up to 100 AUD per spin on a multi-terminal gambling machine in Australian clubs. It is easy to lose an average 1,200 AUD per hour on poker machines in Australian clubs and hotels (Livingstone 2005).

The changing structure of the gambling industry

There have been significant changes in the gambling market's structure in recent years. One example is the casino sector. The US gambling market, still the world's largest in absolute size at a GGR of approximately 94 billion EUR in 2016 (The Economist 2017), is shifting from Nevada (primarily Las Vegas) to other states. Pennsylvania and New Jersey (Atlantic City) are now the second and third most popular casino destinations. There have been heavy investments in casinos in Ohio, New York, Connecticut, and Maryland as these states have moved to attract gambling revenue to their jurisdictions. In Nevada itself, non-gambling revenue (hotels, restaurants, etc.) is increasingly important, since it forms 60% of the total revenue produced on "The Strip" in Las Vegas. This is a remarkable change from 40% in 2005.

After a five-fold increase that began in 2006, the Asia-Pacific region today has joined North America in dominating the global casino market, at an estimated GGR of 64 billion EUR. The Asia-Pacific market is dominated to a considerable extent by Australia and China, two countries whose cultures are congenial to gambling, though casinos remain forbidden in mainland China. Europe and Latin America were estimated to produce GGR of 18.3 billion and 4.5 billion EUR, respectively, in the same year.

The structure of the gambling industry varies by country and region, but one general trend is concentration of ownership into a small number of individuals, families, and corporations. Ownership in the United States is heavily concentrated in a few large Las Vegas and East Coast operators. The leading casino company in the world is Las Vegas Sands, with a turnover of 11.7 billion EUR in profits in 2014. Most of the 12 largest casino companies, including MGM Resorts and Caesar's Entertainment, are US-based. Three (SJM, Galaxy, and Melco Crown) have their headquarters in Hong Kong, the financial center adjacent to Macau. These companies are profitable. In 2013, stock price gains in the Dow Jones US Gaming Index more than doubled the performance of the Standard & Poor's 500 (S & P 500), the leading indicator of US equities, incorporating the 500 largest companies and approximately 80% of US market capitalization. The 11 most exchanged gambling companies in the United States generated an average return of 65.7% compared to the 29.0% return of the S &

P 500 in a similar period. Seven out of the 11 major gambling companies generated returns of over 70%, high for any investment.

UK gambling operators William Hill and Ladbrokes have developed a strong presence in various markets internationally, including Europe and Australia. UK-headquartered companies, often operating through low-tax jurisdictions outside the EU, are major players in growing markets in internet and other remote forms of gambling, but they also operate land-based sites. A report for the European Union notes that UK bookmakers William Hill and Ladbrokes have clients in over 150 and 160 countries, respectively. Ladbrokes offers remote gambling services in 11 languages. Another UK-based company, Expekt.com, moved from London to Malta in 2000. It serves internet customers from 227 countries using 19 languages, mainly focused on the Scandinavian market. The leading pan-European sportsbook is an Austrian-based bookmaker, Win2Day, operating out of Gibraltar under UK jurisdiction. The leading global mobile gambling company is Sportingbet, UK-based but operating from Antigua. Others include companies such as Betfred (United Kingdom), Punt Club (Australia, a social betting service), Openbet (United Kingdom), Unibet, and 888 Holdings (Gibraltar).

Some jurisdictions have established monopolies licensed to be the sole providers, or operated directly by the state. State lotteries with exclusive operating rights have been common in Europe and North America in the 19th and 20th centuries. State monopolies account for 20% of online gambling in Europe, the share being much higher in Northern Europe than in Southern or Eastern Europe. Many countries that have had a government-owned gambling monopoly are privatizing, collecting the public revenue in the form of taxes and other payments from licensed private companies. For example, The Netherlands restructured its gambling framework in 2015. Even the Nordic countries, a traditional stronghold of state monopolies, are increasingly privatizing, Denmark having the most liberal licensing framework. Outside of Europe, Australia provides perhaps the clearest illustration of the privatization of gambling operations, as described in Box 3.3.

Growth of online and mobile gambling

A major change that has occurred since the mid-1990s is a growing tendency to use computers and handheld devices to place bets. This has created a situation in which gambling is available 24 hours a day and practiced without entering a venue. The volume of online gambling increased fourfold between 2004 and 2017. Close to one half of the global online revenue is produced in Europe (Ahmed 2017). Several new actors have emerged to conduct operations

Box 3.3 Privatization and the dynamics of gambling in Australia

Most legal gambling in Australia was operated by state-owned Totalisator Agency Boards (TABs), originally focused on betting on horse races, until 1970. Since that time, gambling activities have gradually been privatized, and also substantially deregulated. State governments rely on gambling taxes and licensing fees to cover the cost of public services, as they have limited ability to raise revenues otherwise. For example, the Victorian government signed an agreement in 2014, an election year, with James Packer's Crown Casino to extend its license to 2050, and to substantially increase the numbers of EGMs and table games in the casino, in return for payments including an immediate contribution of 250 million AUD. The agreement includes provision for compensation to Crown Casino if future governments impose harm prevention restrictions, or an end to the exemption allowing indoor tobacco smoking in the casino's high-stakes gambling areas (Savage 2014; Victorian Responsible Gambling Foundation 2014).

Australia has one of the highest per capita gambling losses in the world. Approximately six billion AUD (3.5 billion EUR in 2015) of the losses are collected by state governments via license fees and taxes. The balance of gambling losses, 15 billion AUD (8.8 billion EUR), is shared among private enterprises and 6,500 registered and licensed not-for-profit clubs (e.g., golf, football), employing close to 100,000 people (in a country of 24.5 million people). A large part of the gambling licensed to clubs is operated by large private companies. Club gambling revenue is intended to be for charitable purposes, but only a minor share of these proceeds are donated (Markham and Young 2014).

Privatization and deregulation have generated substantial wealth for some individuals. One of Australia's richest persons, James Packer, inherited his fortune but then invested it in gambling businesses, including casinos and an online operator, CrownBet. These businesses generated 490 million AUD (290 million EUR) profit in 2013. In 2014 the personal wealth of Packer was 7.7 billion AUD (4.5 million EUR). Len Ainsworth founded Aristocrat Leisure Ltd, a manufacturer of EGMs and other gambling-related technology, and is currently the Chief Executive Officer of Ainsworth Game Technology. With the success of these companies, Ainsworth has been able to generate family wealth of 1.5 billion AUD (0.9 billion EUR). Aristocrat and Ainsworth together sold 300 million AUD worth of EGMs in Australia

> **Box 3.3 Privatization and the dynamics of gambling in Australia**
> *(continued)*
>
> in 2012–13. Others who have profited from gambling privatization and deregulation in Australia are hotel and pub owners, and those running smaller gambling operations. These include Centrebet founded by the Kafartaris family, the former Sportsbet owner Matthew Tripp, and The Australian Leisure and Hospitality Group, of which Woolworths Ltd, a major grocery chain, owns 75%. All these groups have assets over 100 million AUD (59 million EUR) (Markham and Young 2014).

offshore without necessarily having bricks-and-mortar gambling venues at all. This has produced a response from more established gambling operators, who are expanding their range of products to include online operations.

The largest online company in the world in 2016 was Paddy Power Betfair PLC. Three quarters of its revenues are obtained from international markets (Ahmed 2017). The company paid its CEO Denise Coates a record-high salary of 199 million GBP in 2016, and she is now the highest-paid executive in the United Kingdom (Christie 2017). The success of online gambling companies located in Ireland and the United Kingdom is partly due to the fact that China, India, and the United States restrict the activity. Thus online gambling companies seek growth from "grey markets", such as Turkey and Malaysia, where regulation of gambling is less restrictive (Ahmed 2017).

The total market in GGR was 9.4 billion EUR in Italy in 2015 for legal online gambling alone (iGaming Business 2015), and it is the second largest market in online gambling in 2016 (Stradbrooke 2017). Illegal gambling in Italy is remarkable, 1.3 billion EUR (The Guardian 2014). The United Kingdom has the largest online gambling market in Europe with a GGR of 13.6 billion GBP per year. Based on a licensing system, it accounted for 32% of the total gambling market (Gambling Commission UK, n.d.). This is a signifcant proportion given that in Europe online gambling was only approximately 17% of the market share in 2015 (EGBA 2016).

Conclusion

Trends over the past 50 years, and especially in the first two decades of the 21st century, indicate a growing commercialization of gambling, the development of new technologies, a globalization of the market, and the concentration of many gambling activities into arrangements between large transnational corporations and governments. Traditional forms of gambling have been modernized, and new opportunities have been added in the form of internet gambling.

The United States had for decades been the leading legal gambling market, but North America has been eclipsed by Asia Pacific countries in per capita levels and total volumes. Markets in Europe and Latin America have grown more moderately, and Africa remains at a low level.

The expansion of the gambling market has been made possible by political decisions to remove or relax restrictive regulation of the market in many countries. Hardly any cases can be found where legitimate growth in this sector has been possible without legislative change. Availability of online gambling is often used as the justification for increasing liberalization of gambling laws, but it is important to point out that the policy-related gambling expansion started well before the internet became a major platform for the activity at the turn of the millennium. A factor more directly related to the expansion is the neoliberal turn. This commenced about 1980, the time when world financial markets began to be deregulated. A key factor leading to liberalization has been governments' need for funding under conditions where they have been reluctant or unable to rely on taxes from other economic activities.

During the 20th century, the major justification for legal gambling was the collection of money for charitable or governmental purposes by lotteries, or taxes on sports betting (Jensen 2017). Today gambling has become a major industry with global dimensions, operated mostly by international companies, especially in the casino sector and on the internet (Markham and Young 2015). A shrinking proportion of the legal gambling market is operated by state owned companies.

International trade organizations and the European Union have taken an interest in gambling markets, but only after their expansion had already begun. Their interests, as well as the emphasis in many governments' gambling policies, have been in gaining control of illegal markets, preventing tax evasion, establishing equal treatment of competing market actors, and promoting fair consumer policy.

A striking feature of the modern trends in liberalization and privatization is not only the concentration of the industry, but also the concentration of the profits in a small number of families and/or corporations, as well as increasing dependence of state actors on revenues from gambling proceeds. A second feature is the increasing availability of gambling through the internet and EGMs to large segments of the population. As we will show in later chapters, a large proportion of losses are derived from those least able to afford this recreational activity, which for some becomes an extremely expensive diversion. For many, this is now also a life-threatening addiction.

Chapter 4

The range and burden
of gambling problems

A public interest approach must assess the global expansion of gambling in the light of the whole range of its problematic consequences, not only those experienced by the gambling individuals themselves. Besides addiction, these include financial problems as well as physical and mental health issues that are usually experienced as a burden by the gambler's family, social networks, and the communities they live in. The term "harmful gambling" encompasses all degrees of severity and frequency, including "problem" and "pathological" gambling. Gambling behavior itself does not need to be problematic to cause harm. Research has connected gambling to criminality, as well as other societal impacts ranging from cultural harm to environmental questions. Inequality is an issue that deserves special attention.

In this chapter, we discuss the diverse problems—for individuals, families, communities, and society—which are associated with gambling. We outline the nature and extent of the problems, and consider aggregate cost-benefit analyses (CBA) that have been applied to them.

Main categories of gambling problems

An Australian study (Victorian Competition and Efficiency Commission 2012) identified four categories of problems for the gambler at the individual or interactional level: financial, mental health, physical health, and crime. The following summary gives the percentages of clients who reported having experienced each type of issue when they contacted Australian counseling agencies for gambling problems:

- Financial problems: financial loss (64%), job adversely affected (55%), lost job (19%)

- Relationship and family problems: break-up of partners (26%), borrowing from household money (34%)

- Criminal behavior: obtaining money illegally (42%), trouble with police (18%)

- Addiction and mental health problems: would have liked to stop but couldn't (65%), gambled more than intended (83%), depression (96%), seriously thought about suicide (58%)

Another Australian study (Dowling et al. 2014) observed that gamblers' "concerned significant others"—mostly partners, but also some family members and friends—who accessed an Australian web-based counseling site reported many of the same problems, such as the family experiencing financial hardship because of the other person's gambling (91%), the quality of the relationship having been affected (96%); stress or anger due to the other person's gambling (98%); and the significant other's physical health having been affected (77%). Along with these individual and relational problems, the Victorian Competition and Efficiency Commission (2012) also identified collective impacts on community character, sense of trust, social participation, and cohesion.

The causal impact of gambling on such problems is often a key issue in considerations of how to minimize them. Particular human behaviors or problems rarely have a single necessary and sufficient cause. More often, the relationship is one of conditional causation: problems occur in combination with multple factors reinforcing one another in a conditional relationship. Heavy gambling might initially be a coping strategy for mental suffering, but other negative consequences are likely to follow from it. These rarely relieve the condition and often aggravate it. Gamblers' and family members' attributions of a problem to gambling are relatively strong evidence, though not determinative, of a causal connection.

Whereas causality may remain in question for some behaviors and problems that co-occur with heavy gambling, there are several types of co-occurring issues that can more firmly be attributed to gambling, most of them directly associated with money problems, harm caused to others, interactional effects, and crime.

Financial harm to the gambler and the gambler's family

Gambling redistributes money. One redistributive effect is from losers to winners, but the main overall net effect is the transfer from players to the game organizers. Game organizers use money to cover costs of the game, to pay employees, to deliver profit to owners, and to produce a surplus that often goes to government budgets or directly to "good causes". Interview studies with problem gamblers reveal that financial problems are among the most pressing unwanted consequences of their participation (Eby et al. 2016; Mathews and Volberg 2013).

Financial harm ranges from gambling away funds intended for household expenditure to unmanageable debt loads and declarations of bankruptcy. The harm usually extends to the household as a whole; often other members of the family are not initially aware that collective resources have been wagered away by the gambler (Borch 2012). Some gamblers and their families may lose all of their valuable possessions, including homes. Others become so preoccupied by gambling that they lose their jobs, causing even more financial difficulty and loss of social status.

Research has found that financial harm is more severe and more prevalent among lower socio-economic groups than among middle or high-income groups (Castrén et al. 2013; Walker et al. 2012). Gambling debts create a variety of problems among indigenous populations (Breen et al. 2011; Schluter et al. 2007). As in the case of health and life-style vulnerability, it is not always possible to establish causality between economic losses and gambling. Common factors, including ill-health and substance use, may underlie both, and poverty may lead to problematic gambling and vice versa. In any case, gambling always aggravates poverty. Table 4.1 provides estimates of the financial harm of gambling in the Australian population.

Table 4.1 Financial gambling-related harm reported by non-problem gamblers, problem gamblers, and problem gamblers in counseling.

Financial harms from gambling	% Non-problem gamblers	% Problem gamblers (SOGS 5+)[1]	% Problem gamblers in counseling (SOGS 5+)[1]
Owed money to pay for gambling	4.6	51.4	n/a
Borrowed money without paying back	0.7	18.7	53
Borrowed from loan sharks	0.1	5.8	8.4
Declared bankruptcy	0.03	1.4	8.4
Sold property to gamble	0.3	10.8	36.7
Lost a house	n/a	n/a	7.9
Used pawnbrokers to get funds to gamble	0.5	13.1	n/a

[1] SOGS 5+ means a score of 5 or more on the South Oaks Gambling Scale (see Chapter 5), which is indicative of problem gambling.

Reprinted from Productivity Commission 2010, Gambling, Report no. 50, Canberra (https://www.pc.gov.au/inquiries/completed/gambling-2009/report/gambling-report-volume1.pdf) under the CC BY 3.0 AU license.

The data in Table 4.1 is somewhat dated; a more recent study made in Queensland (Queensland Government Treasury 2007) found that almost 40% of persons classified as problem gamblers reported that gambling had adversely affected their job performance and almost 15% had changed jobs for this reason. More than half said that their gambling had sometimes caused financial problems for the household.

Gambling-related debt and poverty

Gambling is a significant contributor to individual debt and both transient and persistent poverty (Barnard et al. 2014). Gambling-related debt occurs when borrowed money is spent on gambling, or when individuals and families are obliged to borrow money to meet financial commitments created by gambling losses (Downs and Woolrych 2010).

Problem gamblers often have debts. Studies conducted in the United States, (Grant et al. 2010), Canada (Williams et al. 2011a), and Australia (Australian Productivity Commission 1999) have found significant average current debts per problem gambler, with estimates ranging from USD 2,500 to over USD 53,000 depending on the sample. These figures are only suggestive as the methods differ across studies, do not consider illegally obtained debts, and are based mostly on gamblers' self-reports (Downs and Woolrych 2009). But not all problem gamblers incur debts, and a third factor may explain the link when it does exist.

The severity of the gambling problem is positively associated with amount of debt (Gerstein et al. 1999). Some games generate more debt than others. In one study of treatment-seeking pathological gamblers (Petry 2003), EGM players had higher current and lifetime debts than average, while players of scratch tickets and lotteries had lower debt levels.

Some studies suggest that gambling is a direct cause of indebtedness (Brown et al. 2012; Downs and Woolrych 2009), and debt may also serve as a motivator to continue playing (Karter 2013; Chun et al. 2011). The least advantaged experience financial stress, job insecurity, and other forms of deprivation that are further exacerbated by gambling (Tu et al. 2014). As a result, gambling-related problems accumulate in the very populations that have the most limited means to face them.

Personal bankruptcy

Some problem gamblers may be obliged to declare bankruptcy in the face of a hopeless financial situation. Personal bankruptcy is not an option in all jurisdictions, and most evidence comes from the United States. A substantial proportion of problem gamblers report having declared bankruptcy; lifetime prevalence is around 10% to 20% (Grant et al. 2010; Komoto 2014). Thus, personal bankruptcy is more prevalent among problem gamblers than among other gamblers and non-gamblers. Among problem gamblers, bankruptcy is often reported as due to gambling, and is associated with other problems in the legal, family, and mental health domains (Grant et al. 2010).

An association between gambling and personal bankruptcy is observed also at the community level; US counties and cities with major gambling facilities have significantly higher bankruptcy filing rates than counties without gambling (Goss and Morse 2005). It has been argued that such co-variation in gambling availability and bankruptcy rates may be due to differences in bankruptcy laws (Gerstein et al. 1999) or establishment of casinos in economically deprived areas (De la Viña and Berstein 2002). However, studies have in most cases found that introduction of casino or other forms of gambling in a community increased the rates of personal bankruptcies (Williams et al. 2011b).

Homelessness

Problem gambling can affect housing stability, and lead to homelessness, i.e., living in shelters, on the streets, or in transient situations such as in a car or in abandoned buildings (Gattis and Cunningham-Williams 2011). A number of studies carried out with homeless individuals either seeking treatment or recruited in the streets have found co-occurring problematic gambling (Sharman et al. 2015; Dufour et al. 2014; Crane et al. 2005). In a three-nation study of the United Kingdom, the United States, and Australia, an average of 15% of homeless respondents reported having gambling problems, with an exceptionally high proportion (39%) registered in Melbourne (Crane et al. 2005). Gambling can be a risk factor for homelessness, and homeless individuals often cite gambling as at least a partial reason for their lack of housing (Holdsworth and Tiyce 2013). Studies have particularly connected bookmakers and amusement arcade EGM gambling to homeless gambling (Sharman et al. 2015).

Work-related problems and job loss

Gambling-related problems may spill over to reduced work performance and absenteeism, and in some cases to job loss (Eby et al. 2016; Williams et al. 2011b).

Online gambling during work time causes productivity losses, money borrowing from colleagues, and requests for cash advances on salary (Griffiths 2009). Gambling may even encourage criminal acts, including embezzlement, stealing goods at work or fraudulent expense claims (Downs and Woolrych 2009). These impacts are particularly important at gambling venues. Employees of the gambling sector have higher rates of problem gambling either because they increase their gambling after being employed in the sector, or because people with a pre-existing attraction to gambling seek employment in the sector (Guttentag et al. 2012; Hing and Breen 2008).

Harm to families and concerned significant others

Problems from gambling are seldom limited to the individual alone. For every problem gambler, a number of other people are also affected. Estimates vary widely depending on definitions and methods of measurement. It is safe to say that on average at least six other persons will be affected, the highest estimates going up to 17 (Kalischuk et al. 2006). In any case, concerned significant others (CSO) form a greater proportion of the population than problem gamblers themselves. General population surveys have found CSO prevalence rates between 2% and 20% (Salonen et al. 2014). High levels of gambling-related harm are reported by intimate partners, parents, siblings, friends, and the extended family, including grandparents, cousins, aunts, or brothers/sisters-in-law (Dowling 2014; Dowling et al. 2014; Valentine and Hughes 2010; McComb et al. 2009). In an Australian sample of help-seekers (Dowling et al. 2014), female partners formed the majority of concerned significant others (CSOs), while in a Finnish population study (Salonen et al. 2014), they were most commonly close friends.

Some studies have found that partners of those identified as pathological gamblers experience the consequences of gambling as more severe than the gambler (Ferland et al. 2008). CSOs report gambling-related harm ranging from emotional distress to financial problems and health impacts (Dowling et al. 2014). Gamblers' partners and other significant others themselves have higher levels of alcohol problems, substance abuse, and problem gambling than comparison groups (Wenzel et al. 2008; Dannon et al. 2006), and also are three times more likely to attempt suicide than those in the general population (Lorenz and Yaffee 1989).

The burden of gambling-related problems on families is often made worse by the urgency of the condition. Gambling problems differ from substance abuse in part because they are easier to hide from family members (McComb et al. 2009). Excessive gambling is often only discovered when consequences have become devastating (Borch 2012). Mobile and online technology in particular enables the gambler to play unnoticed (Fulton 2015). Co-occurring substance abuse or mental health problems in problem gamblers may also add to the burden on family members (Velleman et al. 2015).

Family disruption

Problem gamblers have an elevated rate of separation and divorce (Black et al. 2012; Mathews and Volberg 2013; Park et al. 2010). Interview studies with problem gamblers have shown that they are aware of the harm they are causing to their families; they feel guilt and remorse, and want help with a variety of family issues related to marital problems and parenting (Lee 2002; Lorenz and Yaffee 1986).

Families may provide important help for the problem gambler, but this is often at a high emotional and financial cost (Downs and Woolrych 2010). Many partners remain in their unsatisfactory relationships for long periods of time, often to protect the children or to help the gambler (Patford 2009; 2007; Lorenz and Yaffee 1989). Problematic online gambling in particular often remains a secret within the family (Valentine and Hughes 2010). In Asian communities, shame and embarrassment related to gambling may further increase these difficulties. Asian families, including extended families, are routinely mobilized to bear the burden of problem gambling instead of seeking professional help (Mathews and Volberg 2013; Scull and Woolcock 2005).

Harm to children

The effects of parental gambling on children can be significant (Darbyshire et al. 2001). In addition to economic difficulties due to parental gambling, children can suffer long-term effects of prolonged neglect and uninvolved parenting (Velleman et al. 2015; Darbyshire et al. 2001). Children of problem gambling parents have an elevated risk of physical and mental health problems and suicide attempts (Black et al. 2015; Vitaro et al. 2008; Oei and Raylu 2004). Moreover, these children have a poor quality of life and problems with school work and the legal system (Jacobs et al. 1989; Vander Bilt and Franklin 2003). Children of problem gamblers are more likely than average to develop gambling problems of their own (Dowling et al. 2010) as well as other risky behaviors such as substance use or sexual promiscuity (Dowling et al. 2010; Oei and Raylu 2004). The association between parental problem gambling and harm to children may be exacerbated in remote areas and among indigenous and other minority populations (Stevens and Bailie 2012).

Domestic violence

Domestic violence associated with gambling is an extreme form of harm to families. A meta-analysis shows that a third of problem gamblers report perpetrating intimate partner violence and a similar proportion report being victims of intimate partner violence (Dowling et al. 2016). Gambling-related domestic violence is more common in Asian than in western countries and among Asian communities living abroad (see Keen et al. 2015). Pathological gambling has also been connected to homicide in the family (Wong et al. 2014; Anderson et al. 2011).

As with other co-occurring problems, the association between problem gambling and domestic violence is complex. Gambling has been found to be both its cause and a consequence (Dowling et al. 2016).

Gambling and crime

Gambling is associated with crime in many ways. Individuals may commit crimes in order to get resources for gambling or to pay for gambling losses. The provision of illegal gambling is widespread in many parts of the world, as discussed in Chapter 3, and fraud is common especially in sports. Casinos and online gambling sites offer possibilities for organized and professional criminals to commit illegal acts such as money laundering. Other criminal activities are frequently associated with gambling, including prostitution, drug trading, and illegal (online) pornography. Gambling destinations attract street crime, and alcohol served in gambling venues increases alcohol-related crimes such as driving under the influence of alcohol and drugs (Williams et al. 2011b).

Crime committed by gamblers

Problem and pathological gamblers are more likely to commit crimes than other people in the general population (Cook et al. 2015; Laursen et al. 2016; Williams et al. 2011b). The national community survey (n = 3,498) conducted in Australia by the Australian Productivity Commission (1999) found that 27% of those with severe gambling problems reported having committed crimes related to their gambling during their lifetime. Studies of clinical samples report rates of up to 30% with past year offences (Spapens 2008a). Levels of problem gambling have also been high in forensic populations. A review showed that on average 33% of criminal offenders meet criteria for pathological gambling, and an average of 50% of their crimes are committed to support gambling (Williams et al. 2005).

Problem gamblers commit crimes related to child abuse, family violence, and illegal drugs as has been discussed in this chapter, but also economic crimes, such as tax evasion, fraud, false insurance claims, and embezzlement or theft from family or work (Lind et al. 2015; Laursen et al. 2016; Williams et al. 2011b). A Finnish study of suspected crimes related to gambling (Kuoppamäki et al. 2014) found that these were typically minor financial crimes (64% of the cases), but also other crimes were relatively frequent. In 16% of the cases, the gambler was the victim. Gamblers commit crimes in gambling both online and in real world venues (Banks 2014; McMullan and Rege 2010; Smith et al. 2003) and 'silent' crimes such as stealing from family members (Huberfeld and Dannon 2014).

Different types of gambling attract different types and amounts of criminal offences. Smith et al. (2003) found that few crimes are associated with low-intensity gambling such as lotteries or sports betting. High-intensity gambling modes, such as EGMs, have the most potential to cause problem gambling, and by extension, gambling-related crimes.

Gambling and crime at the community level

A significant body of work compares crime rates before and after a new gambling opportunity has been introduced in a community. The bulk of this research is focused on US casinos. Evidence has been mixed; most studies have found some increase in crime, primarily in assault and property offences, particularly fraud, embezzlement, theft, and larceny, but there are also a number of comprehensive, well conducted studies that found very little or no impact of gambling introduction on crime (Williams et al. 2011b; Humphreys and Soebbing 2014).

The link between gambling and crime may also apply to other gambling opportunities than casinos. An Australian study compared rates of EGM expenditure and crime in Victoria's local areas in 1996, 2001, and 2006 (Wheeler et al. 2010). Results showed a significant relationship between EGM expenditures and crime, especially for income-generating crimes.

Critics have attributed increasing crime rates to increases in population size and tourism (Reece 2010; Baxandall and Sacerdote 2005). Even so, this means that the increase in revenues from tourism is not a benefit without problems. Crime may also increase with a time lag, explaining why some impact studies have found no effect (Williams et al. 2011b).

Organized and professional crime

The most common form of professional or organized crime linked to gambling is illegal supply, frequently used as an argument to liberalize gambling laws (Ferentzy and Turner 2009; Marshall 2009). Nevada had a large amount of illegal gambling before the legalization of casinos in 1931, but the underground market has since disappeared (Thompson 2010). Organized crime continues to be involved in casino and gambling operations in geographical areas such as Southern Italy, Russia, and China (Wang and Antonopoulos 2015). The internet has increased the foothold of illegal gambling opportunities. Online gambling can take place in jurisdictions where it is illegal, underage players can make bets, or operators may not have a license (Banks 2014). The remote (online) gambling industry is very fluid. Operators can easily move to countries with looser regulations. Criminals can therefore operate from jurisdictions that do not screen their backgrounds (Spapens 2014). Illegal and unlicensed operators do not pay taxes or other fees while diverting consumption from the legal market. The European Commission (2012) has estimated that 38% to 90% of online gambling in European markets is unregulated.

Other crimes occur within the legal gambling framework, such as match-fixing, money laundering, and extorting or cheating with counterfeit chips or by rigging EGMs (Spapens 2008a). Boundaries between legal and illegal markets are blurred. Organized crime has a major interest in all forms of gambling: legal, para-legal, and illegal. First, the legal gambling market represents a major opportunity for organized crime to recycle and reinvest money obtained through traditional criminal activities, for instance by purchasing with additional charge winning lottery tickets. Furthermore, illegal organizations penetrate the gambling market in different ways, which, based on police investigations, include extortions imposed on concessionaires and gambling venues; pressures on managers of public premises to install video poker machines; infiltration into the legal market by either dummies or shareholding; and the management of unauthorized betting on websites located in foreign countries (Anti-Mafia Commission 2016).

Online environments offer many opportunities for manipulating games, and for using players' credit cards and account information to skim funds or to commit identity fraud (Spapens 2014). Fraudulent sites take customers' money but do not pay winnings. Typical cases have involved fake lotteries (Griffiths 2010; McMullan and Rege 2010). Criminals may also create forgeries of legitimate sites (Banks 2014), and hackers may steal players' personal information (McMullan and Rege 2010). A new form of criminality has been cyber-extortion of online gambling providers. According to an online analysis conducted by McMullan and Rege (2010), hundreds of gambling websites have been subject to such attacks.

Money laundering is recognized as an issue in gambling legislation in many jurisdictions (Spapens 2008a), while match-fixing has been particularly pervasive in Asia (Spapens 2014). There is also some evidence that even legal gambling can have a corrupting influence on police and politicians. Lobbying, bribery, and subtle contributions to public officials have been used to promote laws permitting the establishment of casinos (Pontell et al. 2014; Campbell et al. 2005). Panel data from US states between 1985 and 2000 (Walker and Calcagno 2013) found that once casinos are established, they tend to influence politicians to push for further deregulations.

Gambling regimes as drivers of social inequality

The more that gambling opportunities are created, the more social inequality is likely to increase. Higher-income households have on average higher spending on gambling in absolute terms than poorer households, but poorer households lose a higher proportion of their income on gambling, and do not have the financial resources to buffer the losses (Lang and Omori 2009). Thus gambling revenues are often called 'regressive taxation'. A counter-argument is that gambling expenditures are voluntary expenditures. While this reasoning may be applicable to the gambler, there is often no voluntary choice to family members or others whose finances are linked to the gambler.

An interview study from Germany (Beckert and Lutter 2009) (n = 1,508) showed that the lowest income quintile spends an average of 12% of their net income on gambling, compared to only 2% in the highest quintile. The same study showed that 50% of gambling turnover is borne by just 12.6% of all gamblers. Similar figures have been obtained elsewhere. Data from combined 2008 and 2009 population surveys conducted in Alberta, Canada, found that 5.8% of the population account for 75% of reported gambling expenditure. The top 20% of spenders account for 89.1% of all gambling spending (Williams et al. 2011a); see also Chapter 6. These figures are based on cross-sectional data at a particular point in time, and they do not account for the turnover of the low income heavy players: those at the peak of gambling expenditure are unlikely to be able to continue their pattern of expenditure after they have run through their stock of credit and fiduciary relationships. The fluidity of the top of the gambling distribution, and the large number of persons affected by unbearable losses, mean that the actual prevalence of people whose life chances have been hurt by gambling is much greater than cross-sectional prevalence figures based on individual data suggest.

Social inequality in gambling differs somewhat according to the game in question. Lottery participation is highest among those with low socioeconomic status (Papineau et al. 2015; Crowley et al. 2013; Beckert and Lutter 2009). Clotfelter et al. (1999) found that low income groups in the United States actually spent more money on the lottery in both absolute and relative terms than high income groups. EGM gambling has also been connected to low socioeconomic status (Schissel 2001). Availability and active encouragement of EGM gambling among less wealthy populations in the most deprived neighborhoods (Wardle et al. 2014; Wheeler et al. 2006) contribute to this effect. Pearce et al. (2008) have calculated that the median travel distance to the closest EGM in deprived areas is about half of the distance in more privileged areas. Internet gambling forms an exception to the general rule, as online players tend to be more highly educated and have higher incomes than gamblers who do not play on the internet (Tovar et al. 2013; Williams et al. 2011a).

The disproportionately high spending by low-income groups both in relative and in some cases absolute terms means that the money collected from players aggravates inequality and forms a poverty spiral. Several mechanisms contribute to the spiral. First, gambling expenditures have direct income transfer effects from the poor to the more wealthy (Freund and Morris 2006). In the media and elsewhere, gambling revenues are often referred to as a regressive tax, and empirical evidence supports this. A statistical analysis of gambling expenditures conducted in Australia (Worthington 2001) showed that gambling-related taxation is regressive, even when other factors such as household income sources and welfare benefits were taken into account. Another study, conducted in Texas (Price and Novak 1999), concluded that taxation of lottery tickets is more regressive than another regressive form of taxation, the Value Added Tax (a sales tax).

The second mechanism is that among lower income groups, a high proportion of income spent on gambling often leads to financial problems (Freund and Morris 2006; Welte et al. 2004b), as they are less likely to have the necessary financial resources to buffer gambling losses. This may lead to taking out loans, including expensive unsecured loans. As a result, gambling-related problems accumulate in the very populations that have the most limited means to face them. A longitudinal study based on state-level data from the United States on income inequality and gambling expenditures (1980–1997) found that greater income inequality increases the average expenditure on gambling (Bol et al. 2014). How strong a driver gambling is of inequality depends on return rates and the proportion of participants who belong to low income groups. This varies between countries and games, the United States showing higher income regressivity than other countries (Beckert and Lutter 2009).

Economic downturns may strengthen the relationship between gambling and income inequality. A time-series analysis of over 50 years of data in the United States has shown that spending on lotteries is maintained or increased during recessions (Horváth and Paap 2012). A New Zealand study (Tu et al. 2014) examined the impact of the financial crisis on gambling expenditures. Using representative health surveys conducted in 2008, 2010, and 2012, the study found that although overall gambling participation had dropped, households were experiencing more gambling-related harm in 2012 compared with the earlier years. Residents of more deprived areas were 4.5 times more likely to experience gambling-related problems than those from wealthier neighborhoods.

One explanation put forward to explain why economically deprived populations tend to gamble to their disadvantage is that gambling offers to many the only perceived possibility of escaping poverty, feeding aspirations for social mobility or access to consumer goods (Beckert and Lutter 2009; Schissel 2001). Other explanations include greater financial risk-taking relative to income (Tabri et al. 2015; Bol et al. 2014; Callan et al. 2008, 2011); that gambling offers stress relief (Bol et al. 2014; Nibert 2000); and that poor gamblers may not be aware of the redistributive mechanisms and outcomes of the activity (Rogers 1998; Rogers and Webley 2001).

Social costs of gambling studies and cost-benefit models

The impact of gambling on societies depends on a number of factors, including types of games and gambling environments that are available, how long gambling has been available, the effectiveness of policy interventions, and how gambling revenue is ultimately distributed (Williams et al. 2011b). In most jurisdictions, and in most time periods, the impacts of gambling have been mixed, with some mild positive but also negative social impacts (Williams et al. 2011b). Political decision makers tend to rely on cost-benefit estimates, but there is no scientific consensus on how such estimates should be calculated, and the available research is of varying quality.

The overall socioeconomic impact of gambling can be evaluated from a cost of illness (COI) perspective, adapted from the public health field. Such studies have been common in alcohol and drug research, but this perspective does not consider the benefit side (Walker 2007). Economic cost-benefit analysis (CBA), applied in a variety of environmental and infrastructure policy issues, constructs aggregate balance sheets of tangible costs and benefits to evaluate alternative plans (Walker 2007). This approach requires that a monetary value is also assigned to intangible harm and the harm that that accrues to other people and to society at large, besides the gamblers themselves. Most of the harms caused by gambling that have been discussed in this chapter are of this nature. The utility of this approach is disputed. In their review, Williams et al. (2011b) stated that it is a mistake to try to capture social impacts that do not have significant monetary consequences within a cost-benefit economic framework by applying an arbitrary monetary value to them. They further argue that "this approach fails to recognize that the true nature of the impact is largely non-monetary in nature" (Williams et al. 2011b). Nevertheless, some studies have applied this approach. Obviously, different definitions of the entries as well as decisions on causal attribution determine the estimates produced. The Australian Productivity Commission (2010; 1999) conducted a comprehensive large-scale calculation including bankruptcy, productivity loss, crime, legal costs, personal and family problems, divorce, violence, depression, suicide, and treatment. Depression was estimated to be the biggest burden in monetary terms. The Commission's 1999 report concluded that gambling created a loss for society, but the more recent report (2010) estimated the net benefit to the community to range between 3.7 and 11.1 billion AUD. Gaming machines caused the biggest costs, followed by wagering bets, while lotteries and scratch tickets had notably lower cost estimates.

In Sweden, the total national costs on health, social control, treatment, and social services excluding family disruption and crime have been estimated to be approximately 250–485 million EUR per year, while the net profit of the monopoly operator Svenska Spel is approximately 540 million (Svenska Spel 2011).

The National Gambling Impact Study in the United States estimated that in 1998 the annual cost per problem gambler (due to job loss, unemployment benefits, welfare benefits, poor physical and mental health, and treatment) amounted to approximately 900 USD, being considerably lower than estimated annual costs per case in several other health problem areas, such as drug abuse, alcohol abuse, and mental illness (Gerstein et al. 1999). This estimate did not include the lifetime costs related to bankruptcy, arrests, imprisonment, and legal fees. Nor did it take into account organized crime, corruption and theft related to gambling, and more indirect costs related to family members. These less tangible social and individual costs cannot be given a monetary value.

The Victorian Competition and Efficiency Commission (2012) estimated that the total social and economic cost of problem gambling in Victoria including quantifiable and intangible costs was between 1.4 billion and 2.7 billion USD (approximate equivalent of AUD) in 2010–2011, representing approximately 45,000 to 85,000 USD per problem gambler per year. A more recent study put this cost at close to 7 billion AUD (Browne et al 2017). The two major contributions to costs were 1) excess expenditure by problem gamblers, which amounts to 50%–65% of the total, and 2) mental ill-health caused to problem gamblers and their families, accounting for 25%–40% of the total.

Different studies have thus come to different conclusions, based on definitional and methodological choices that determine the outcome. A large number of variables with estimated values enter the calculations. Their value for a public interest approach is further reduced by a conceptual issue. The frame is the cost to the society as a whole, but costs and benefits are not equally distributed among individual actors, their social networks, communities, and national or state governments. CBA approaches tend to obscure the reality that in gambling, someone's gain mostly depends on someone else's loss, yet they will be interpreted as balancing each other out.

Conclusion

Substantial evidence links gambling with individual and social harms in health, poverty, social relationships, and crime. Gambling is a co-occurring problem among people who are already in vulnerable life situations. It aggravates their difficulties and obstructs their attempts to improve their situation. The relation between gambling and life difficulties of the vulnerable is multifactorial, perhaps the result of conditional causation rather than a matter of a single cause. This is particularly the case in the literature on comorbidity, referring to the fact that a very large percentage of problem and pathological gamblers also have mental and physical health problems, problems with substance use, or both.

In the types of harmful consequences discussed in this chapter the causal link is more obvious or probable. This is true of economic losses, of damage in intimate relationships, and of some forms of crime. These are harms caused to the social entourage rather than only to the gambling individuals themselves. In policy terms, this invites consideration of social utility in a perspective wider than eliminating or reducing the risk of problem and pathological gambling behavior.

Available socioeconomic impact studies applying the cost-benefit approach are based on limited geographic areas, and they have been unable to account for the fact that costs and benefits of gambling fall on different parties, often those who do not participate in gambling at all. Gambling undeniably increases inequality. The number of individuals who produce the most part of the total wager, of the GGR, or of public revenue from gambling, is very small in all societies. The balance of money collected from the activity is a transfer from the poor to the rich. Only in very few cases do poor winners dig their way out by their success. Even considering that a substantial part of the GGR in many countries is returned back to society for good causes that often benefit the poor, gambling revenues to governments are comparable in their income distribution effects to other forms of regressive taxation. This is also the case for national lotteries, which otherwise are less dangerous for participants. Lotteries have very low return percentages, and participation in them is more strongly correlated with low income than other games.

Instead of investing in cost-benefit studies, policymakers should be advised to consider the desired outcomes of gambling separately from its drawbacks. Alternatives to fund-raising for taxes and good causes should be considered.

Indirect and intangible harms and costs to society are subject to too many uncertainties to be assigned precise pecuniary values. Included in these are inequalities, which can be of various kinds, some making the rich even richer, others undermining middle income levels, and yet others aggravating the poverty of those who are already poor. Gambling as a solution to social revenue needs faces the risk of aggravating society's most vexacious social problems by turning poverty into misery, even for many who do not themselves gamble at all.

Chapter 5

Gambling behavior and problem gambling

Gambling is no longer an exclusive activity that only a small number of people engage in. This is especially true in countries where it is legal, accessible, and commercialized. Consistent with data on gambling volumes derived from industry statistics, general population surveys show that gambling is prevalent in many high-income countries, but there are great variations between countries and between sub-populations within countries. From a public interest perspective it is essential to know who are the gamblers, what are the population characteristics underlying within-country differences, and how problem gambling is related to other vulnerabilities.

This chapter describes research on the extent of gambling in different parts of the world, including participation by different population segments in different types of games. Statistical results from population surveys must be interpreted cautiously, keeping in mind important methodological considerations, lest such numbers provide misleading estimates of the gravity of the issue. They do show, however, that a major part of those who suffer from the negative effects of gambling are persons who also suffer from other vulnerabilities.

The prevalence of gambling and its intensity

Few surveys were conducted before the 1980s; 72 were conducted in the 1990s, and between 2000 and 2011 there were 112. In most surveys more than half of the respondents report gambling at least once in the preceding year (Williams et al. 2012a). However, the proportion varies considerably by country and date—between 30% and 90%. Comparisons of survey estimates over time in the small roster of affluent countries which have conducted regular surveys suggest an increase in average past year gambling prevalence from the mid-1970s to 2000, and then a decrease in average past year gambling prevalence over the next decade (Williams et al. 2012a).

Prevalence estimates derived from population surveys (Williams et al. 2012a) roughly correspond to total expenditures, with Australia and Finland having high levels of participation, Italy in the middle, and France and Germany having lower prevalence rates. Surveys in Sweden, the United Kingdom, and Canada show relatively high rates of gambling participation compared with total volumes of losses (Gross Gambling Revenue (GGR)) per resident adult. In contrast, Singapore has the second highest losses per adult resident, but surveys show a rather low participation rate of only 45%, the discrepancy being probably due to the influx of money from abroad in relation to a small population (5.8 million in 2017). The inconsistencies between population surveys and total volumes of GGR also depend on the concentration of gambling in smaller or larger sub-populations, and on the variable quality of the surveys.

The mere prevalence of gambling in a country can be misleading as an exposure measure. Substantial gaps have been found between the prevalence of any gambling in a country, and the prevalence of frequent gambling (Australian Productivity Commission 2010; Costes et al. 2011). These gaps are partly explained by differences in games or modes of gambling (see Box 5.1).

Table 5.1 shows the percentage of respondents in the United Kingdom who reported gambling by type of game in the previous 12 months, and then the proportion of those who gambled in that mode who did it at least once

Box 5.1 Types of game: high- and low-intensity gambling

Game characteristics vary in how much they encourage excessive play. High event frequency, multiple game/stake opportunities, near-misses, stake size, and continuity of play increase the risk of problem gambling (Dowling et al. 2005). Games with these characteristics are called hard or intensive. They include casino games, electronic gambling machines (EGMs), horse and greyhound race betting, as well as instant scratch cards. Soft or low-intensity forms include weekly lotteries and football pools (Griffiths and Wood 2001). The French gambling researcher Marc Valleur (2008) has made similar distinctions based on the stimuli the games produce: 'dream games' (*jeux de rêve*) include lottery type games with low-levels of sensation; 'thrill games' (*jeux de sensation pure*) include EGMs and casino games that involve strong sensations and high intensity levels.

Some games have both high and low intensity characteristics. Operators can change the intensity of the same game in different business hours to optimize returns (Schüll 2012). The technical designs of EGMs differ

---

Box 5.1 Types of game: high- and low-intensity gambling *(continued)*

significantly. In the United States they often provide large top prizes, whereas British variants and Canadian EGMs, called video lottery terminals (VLTs), resemble scratch tickets with small prizes (Rockloff and Hing 2013). Some machines involve real skill elements, such as Japanese pachinko and old European Bajazzo machines (Woolley and Livingstone 2010; Meyer and Bachmann 2011).

The intensity of online gambling is a matter of some disagreement. Online poker has been characterized as only a medium risk game (Clement et al. 2012), but online gambling can simulate nearly any game. Availability, convenience, social isolation, anonymity of participation, electronic payment, higher pay-out rates, and the possibility to play under the influence of alcohol and drugs may make internet gambling more problematic than land-based variants (Wood et al. 2007).

Assessment of the risk potential of various games is often based on general population surveys or studies of help-line callers or gamblers in treatment (Binde 2011; Meyer et al. 2010). Problematic gambling is most often related to EGMs, sports betting, and table games in casinos, but rarely to scratch cards and lotteries (Binde 2011; Meyer et al. 2011). The proportion of problem gamblers is low, even among EGM players (Binde 2011; Lund 2006; Orford et al. 2013). However, problem gamblers account for a disproportionately large fraction of gambling expenditures in casinos and on EGMs. Some variation in problem gambling prevalence over time and between jurisdictions can therefore be attributed to differences in the availability of high intensity games.

---

a week (Wardle et al. 2011a). The majority of respondents who gamble at all participate in lotteries, and these players are likely to do it at least once a week. Instant scratch tickets, horse and dog race betting, and EGMs are also popular, but a smaller proportion of those who are involved in them engage in these games regularly. These are gambling forms where occasional intensive gambling episodes are more characteristic. Similar findings are reported from Australia in 1999 and Victoria in 2003 (Australian Productivity Commission 1999; McMillen et al. 2004a). In France, where EGMs are only available in casinos located mainly in tourist coastal destinations, EGM gambling is less widespread, and intensive EGM gamblers are even more rare (Costes et al. 2015).

Table 5.1 Percentage of adults participating in different types of gambling in the past year, and percentage of participants doing so weekly or more often. The United Kingdom, 2010

Gambling mode	Percent involved in last year	Percent of population participating weekly or more often	Percent of those involved in last year who participate weekly or more often
National Lottery Draw	59	36	61
Another lottery	25	5	20
Scratch cards	24	6	25
Slot machines	13	2	15
Horse races	16	3	19
Bingo	9	3	33
Private betting	11	2	18
Any online gambling	11	5	45
Any gambling	**73**	**43**	**59**

Adapted from Wardle et al (2011) Defining the online gambler and patterns of behaviour integration: evidence from the British Gambling Prevalence Survey 2010. International Gambling Studies 11(3)339-356 with permission from Taylor and Francis.

Demographic characteristics of gamblers

Gender and age

Men gamble more, and play more intensely on more types of games, than women in almost all countries on which data is available. There are some games that women are more likely to play than men, such as scratch cards and bingo (Salonen and Raisamo 2015; Wardle et al. 2011a; Costes et al. 2011; Institut für Therapieforschung 2011; Australian Productivity Commission 1999; IFC-CNR 2014).

Age correlates with gambling participation. Contrary to prevailing images, neither the young nor the old have the highest gambling participation; working age adults have the highest rate (Wardle et al. 2011a, Australian Productivity Commission 1999, Costes et al. 2015, Salonen and Raisamo 2015). Adults aged 45–64 years have the highest proportion of past year gamblers in the United Kingdom (Wardle et al. 2011a), while in France it is adults between 35–54 years (Costes et al. 2015), but the proportion of regular gamblers (at least once a week) increases with age. The preferred game depends on age. Poker and EGMs are most popular with younger age groups, whereas lotteries are more popular in older age groups (e.g., Costes et al. 2011, Salonen and Raisamo 2015, Wardle et al. 2011a). Not surprisingly, online gambling is more common among younger than older age groups (e.g., Wardle et al. 2011b; Costes et al. 2011, IFC-CNR 2014).

Many countries have legal age limits for most types of gambling, but gambling is nevertheless prevalent among adolescents. Young people's initial gambling experiences often occur at home and with family members or peers (Ariyabuddiphongs 2013; Brezing et al. 2010; Raylu and Oei 2002). Early onset of gambling is an important risk factor for problems later in life (Derevensky and Gupta 2000; Rahman et al. 2012). Several studies have found that children of problem gamblers have an elevated risk of problem gambling (Raylu and Oei 2002).

Socio-economic status

Gambling participation varies with socio-economic status. Expenditures in absolute terms tend to increase with income but *expenditures relative to income decrease with increasing income* (Grun and McKeigue 2000; Beckert and Lutter 2009). This means that high-income groups spend more money but low-income groups spend a larger share of their income on gambling. Among heavy users, the amount of money spent does not depend on income: all income categories in the top 25% of gamblers spend large amounts.

Consequently, relative to their income, poor gamblers contribute more to GGR than people with higher income (Williams et al. 2011b). Insofar as the revenue goes to state budgets in the form of taxes and fees, this disproportionate spending is often referred to as *regressive taxation* (Beckert and Lutter 2009; Schissel 2001). Furthermore, there is evidence that the unemployed, the less educated, and low income workers participate more in high intensity games (Albers and Hübl 1997; Wardle et al. 2011a). The unemployed are not necessarily more likely to gamble, but if they do they are often intensive gamblers (Wardle et al. 2011a).

Socio-economic status is also associated with the types of games played. Higher education is a predictor of online gambling participation (e.g., Wardle et al. 2011b), but the demand for lotto tickets is highest among low educational levels and average incomes. The lower middle class with low or average incomes contribute also to state lotteries more than high-income groups, reinforcing the regressive tax effect, if state lotteries are regarded as a 'voluntary tax' for collecting money for state budgets.

Most of the regularities concerning gender, age, and socio-economic status hold generally across populations, but correlations with participation, intensity, and preferred type of gambling depend on the country. For example, the preferred game of women might differ from one country to another, or between ethnic groups even in the same country (e.g., Wardle et al. 2011a; Raylu and Oei 2002). In most countries spending on gambling is higher relative to income among low-income earners, but participation varies by game type.

Stability of gambling behavior over time

Stable patterns of variation in gambling by socio-demographic characteristics in cross-sectional survey studies do not imply stability in individual behavior over time. On the contrary, panel studies following the same individuals suggest that their participation and game preferences change over time. Delfabbro et al. (2009) followed a sample of Australian teenagers from the age of 15 until they reached age 18–19 and found very little stability in game-specific gambling activity. In another longitudinal study from Australia, Delfabbro and colleagues (2014) followed a sample from the age of 16–18 through to the age of 20–21 and found again that relatively few teenagers reported stable patterns, and gambling at age 16–18 was generally not associated with gambling four years later.

What is problem gambling and how is it measured?

Most people gamble without experiencing problems, but some gamble in ways that compromise, disrupt, or damage family, personal, and recreational pursuits (Meyer et al. 2009). Governments often look at estimates of problem gambling in the population when they plan or evaluate changes in gambling regulations.

Terminology concerning problematic gambling behavior varies, reflecting differences in framing the issue. A broad and somewhat imprecise category is *problem gambling* (Williams and Volberg 2014). The term is used in several ways: as a less severe form of gambling disorder than *pathological gambling*, and as a public health term where gambling contributes to various forms of harm (Delfabbro 2013; Williams and Volberg 2014). Definitions of problem gambling are often simplified to mean any gambling that causes harm to the gambler or someone else (Williams and Volberg 2014). Related terms include *compulsive gambling, disordered gambling, excessive gambling*, and *intemperate gambling*. In this book we use *problem* or *problematic gambling* as a generic term. *Gambling disorder, pathological gambling/gambler* and *problem gambling/gambler* will be used when referring to a specific rating scale or diagnostic instrument that is used to provide an operational definition of these terms. Other terms will only be used when referring to a specific source.

The international disease classification and diagnostic systems (i.e., the International Classification of Diseases (World Health Organization, 1993) and the Diagnostic and Statistical Manual of Mental Disorders (American Psychiatric Association 2013)) include *pathological gambling* and *gambling disorder*. Pathological gambling first made its entry into the catalogue of mental disorders as an impulse control disorder (Hodgins et al. 2011), but in the fifth revision of the Diagnostic and Statistical Manual of the American Psychiatric Association (DSM) the term has been altered to *gambling disorder* (Petry et al. 2014). These categories are used for cases where a person reports having experienced a pre-set number of symptoms related to gambling, usually within the past year.

Modified versions of these self-report measurement instruments are used also in general population surveys for prevalence estimates. Individually based survey questions on gambling behavior in the past year, past month, and past two weeks are used to compose summary scales with cut-off points for problem gambling and pathological gambling, depending on the instrument used. These instruments include the *South Oaks Gambling Screen (SOGS)* (Lesieur and Blume 1987); the *Canadian Problem Gambling Index (CPGI)*, the *Problem Gambling Severity Index* (PGSI) (Ferris and Wynne 2001, Holtgraves 2009b), the *Problem and Pathological Gambling Measure (PPGM)* (Williams and Volberg 2010); the *Victorian Gambling Screen (VGS)* (Wenzel et al. 2004); and various diagnostic interviews that are based on DSM or ICD criteria (e.g., *NORC DSM-IV Screen for Gambling Problems (NODS)* (Gerstein et al. 1999).

These instruments contain items that cover in part the same or similar content (*chasing losses, borrowing money for gambling and not paying back*). Some items are particular to one instrument such as *betting more money than one can afford to lose,* and *health or financial problems* (only in PGSI), *theft or embezzlement, spending much time in thinking about gambling, gambling to escape problems and uncomfortable feelings* (only in NODS), or *hiding signs of betting from family and others, gambling more than intended,* and *money arguments centered on betting* (only in SOGS).

Many items familiar from scales on other addictions are included in several but not all instruments. These include *having a problem with money, wanting but unable to stop, feeling guilty, being criticized for gambling, needing to gamble more to have the same effect,* and *lost time from work or school* because of gambling. These differences reflect varying degrees of emphasis on problems caused to others, the role of money, and the nature of the problem as an addiction.

The scales have different maximum scores, and cutting points between moderate, problem, and pathological gambling are comparable only approximately across a continuum of severity. Measures based on screening instruments are easy to administer in population surveys and are commonly used to describe the prevalence of individual gambling problems in different societies (Sassen et al. 2011a).

Limitations of problem gambling prevalence rates

Prevalence rates of problematic gambling found in population studies, however measured, are generally very low, varying from a fraction of a percent to a few percent of the population. As the relative frequencies are low they are very sensitive to errors that can influence the observed rates. For example, a prevalence rate of 1% in a sample of two thousand means twenty people. A random difference of five persons between 20 and 25, who are classified as problem gamblers, means a difference between 1.00% to 1.25%, in other words, a 25% difference in the prevalence rate. Whenever such a difference is observed between two consecutive surveys of the same population, it should not be interpreted as indicating a change in the problem gambling prevalence. Many factors unrelated to real changes in population behavior could have caused the change in the sample: random errors in sample selection, non-response, under- or over-reporting, misunderstandings, and technical errors, just to name a few (Williams et al. 2012a; Walker and Dickerson 1996). Some groups may be excluded altogether from the sampling frame: institutionalized individuals, the homeless, the young, and those who do not have a telephone for various reasons (Williams et al. 2012a; Lesieur 1994). Non-response and refusal bias leave out groups that tend to have higher rates of problem gambling than the general population (Raylu and Oei 2002). These issues are not unfamiliar in population surveys on other behaviors, for example alcohol use (Gmel and Rehm 2004).

The problem gambling assessment instruments that are used (SOGS, DSM, CPGI, NODS, PPGM) give different results (Williams et al. 2012a). Several questions included in the instruments are about social relationships reflecting betrayal of trust, pressure from others hurt by the gambling, and the guilty feelings of the gambler. These questions are culturally sensitive (Abbott and Volberg 1992). Varying cut-off scores on what counts as moderate, problem, or pathological gambling complicate comparisons even more (Sassen et al. 2011a).

Australian studies typically use the SOGS and the CPGI, whereas research conducted in the United States has predominantly used the SOGS and the DSM (Williams et al. 2012a). Since the early 2000s the SOGS has largely been replaced by the CPGI and the DSM (Williams et al. 2012a). Even the same instrument may be applied in different versions and under different names. These limitations must always be kept in mind when comparing survey-based prevalence estimates between countries and especially between two points in time in the same population.

Prevalence of problem gambling

Cross-country variations and overall trends

Prevalence rates of problem gambling range from 0.5% to 7.6% across countries, with an average of 2.3% (Williams et al. 2012a). Most national estimates of problem gambling in the adult population are within the range of 1% to 4% (Williams et al. 2012a), whereas prevalence estimates of pathological gambling are in the range of 0.1% to 0.8% (Bühringer et al. 2013).

Averaged estimates from different studies indicate that problem gambling probably has increased in North America and Australia from the late 1980s to the late 1990s or early 2000s. Thereafter, a downward trend is observed (Williams et al. 2012a). The apparent downward trend is noteworthy, considering the substantial increase in gambling expenditures that occurred simultaneously (see Chapter 3).

The contradiction between declining prevalence rates and simultaneously growing total volume of GGR is in part due to the fact that gaming environments have changed in multiple ways. One example is Switzerland, where observed problem prevalence came down from 2.1% in 1998 to 1.3% in 2005, when new casinos with high spending levels had been opened but EGMs were eliminated at the same time. In Australia, the observed decrease in problem gambling is related to the use of different instruments in later surveys. Thus the results are not directly comparable. In the United States, the decrease in problem gambling is difficult to assess, due to low completion and high refusal rates in population surveys (Welte et al. 2015).

Prevalence rates as measures of the size of the problem

An additional factor, itself of great policy relevance, that needs to be considered in comparisons of prevalence over time, is remission of individuals as they change from problem gamblers to unproblematic players, or to people who cannot continue because they have no money or they are otherwise incapacitated to gamble. Abbot, Williams, and Volberg (2004) found that among current problem and pathological gamblers assessed at one point in time, a third still qualified for these categories after seven years, one half still gambling frequently. A longitudinal study from the United States followed a general population cohort from age 18–19 years to age 29 (Slutske et al. 2003). The problem gambling rate was around 3% and slightly decreased with age, but individual transitions were common. Over the 11 year observation period, 8%

of the sample met criteria for current problem gambling at least once. Life-time problem gambling was considerably more prevalent than current, indicating a great fluidity in the problem gambler population. Such substantial individual transitions are observed also in other areas, as for instance regarding instability in heavy drinking (Skog and Duckert 1993).

As the harms from problem and pathological gambling typically persist for several years, the number of people who are suffering from them at any one time may be significantly higher than what is captured by prevalence rates from population studies (Cassidy et al. 2013; Lesieur 1994). Thus, interpreting changes in such rates over time and from one study to another, even using the same basic methodology, requires careful methodological scrutiny. Given the fact that many people are affected by one problematic gambler, survey-based prevalence rates seriously underestimate the gravity of the issue. Using a broader range of indicators derived from different sources of information (e.g., treatment admissions, helpline calls), and combining survey estimates from several studies, will provide a rough—and probably better—view of how the extent of problem gambling varies.

Demographic characteristics of problem gamblers

Although prevalence rates are weak measures of changes over time, they are useful in showing variations between population segments.

Prevalence of problematic gambling varies with gender and ethnic background in the same way as participation in gambling activities overall. Men are more likely than women to experience problems both in adult general population surveys (Johansson et al. 2009; Petry 2005) and in surveys of adolescent or youth samples (Ariyabuddhiphongs 2013; Blinn-Pike et al. 2010). The male to female ratio varies across studies. In adult population surveys, problem gambling is two to seven times higher among men compared to women (our calculations based on figures in Petry 2005, Table 4.5) and even higher ratios (e.g., 20:1) have been reported (Sassen et al. 2011b). In adolescent populations the prevalence rates are around three to five times higher in males compared to females (Brezing et al. 2010).

In contrast, age variations in experienced gambling problems do not follow the pattern in gambling participation. An early meta-analysis of prevalence rates of pathological gambling among youth in North America (Shaffer and Hall 1996) suggested that these rates were in the range of 4.4% to 7.4%. Other estimates (Derevensky et al. 2003) have been lower, often in the range between 1% and 4% (Volberg et al. 2010). A general finding is that problem gambling is more prevalent in younger age groups compared to middle aged and older persons (Johansson et al. 2009; Petry 2005; Sassen et al. 2011b), whereas the reverse is the case in gambling participation, as noted earlier. A research review (Blinn-Pike et al. 2010) shows that adolescent rates of problem gambling experiences are two to ten times higher than those of adults (based on our calculations and Petry 2005).

Problem gambling rates are often found to be higher in low socio-economic groups, such as the unemployed and persons on welfare, but findings are mixed (Johansson et al. 2009; Petry 2005). Neighborhood disadvantage (e.g., high unemployment, poverty, and households on public assistance) is often associated with problem gambling (Barnes et al. 2013; Martins et al. 2013). This is related to the high density of EGMs and lottery outlets in deprived neighborhoods (Clotfelter and Cook 1991; Gilliland and Ross 2005; Wheeler et al. 2006; Wilson et al. 2006). For example, a US population study (Barnes et al. 2015) showed that the rate of problem gambling was highest (7.5%) in the lowest fifth in socio-economic status, while the lowest rate (1.7%) was found in the highest fifth in socio-economic status. Data from the 2003 British Gambling Prevalence Survey (Orford et al. 2003a) also showed that those in the lowest of three income categories were nearly three times as likely to have gambling problems as the average person, after controlling for other socio-demographic variables.

Problem gambling rates are usually high among ethnic minorities, including indigenous populations (Johansson et al. 2009; Petry 2005; Volberg and Wray 2007; Barnes et al. 2015). For instance, in the United States, Welte and colleagues (2001) found that 11% of Native Americans and 8% of African Americans and Hispanics were problem gamblers as compared to 2% of Caucasian respondents.

Another national survey conducted in the United States (Welte et al. 2002) showed that Native Americans (10.5%), blacks (7.8%), Hispanics (8.0%) and Asians (6.6%) were more likely to be pathological gamblers than whites (1.8%). Similar patterns have been identified among ethnic minorities in other country contexts, such as the Maori and Pacific islanders in New Zealand and recent immigrants in Sweden (Walker et al. 2012; Abbott et al. 2004a). A population study in South Africa (Sharp et al. 2015) found that moderate or high risk gambling was ten times more frequent in the black population (15.1%) than in the white (1.5%). Problem gambling was particularly widespread in mining communities, in which unlicensed taverns and illegal gambling are common. A Canadian population survey (Martins et al. 2010) found a higher proportion of problem gamblers among indigenous Canadians (3.7%) compared to the majority population (0.8%).

Explanations for the higher level of problem gambling in certain popula-tions have been suggested by several investigators. Welte et al. (2004b) showed that ethnic background and socio-economic status influence problem gam-bling even when levels of gambling participation are controlled for. Those having low socio-economic status often see gambling as a means of upward social mobility and as a way to cope with stress. In addition, culture-specific reasons have been identified (e.g., Tepperman and Korn 2004), including cultural variations in motivations and beliefs relevant to gambling (Kim et al. 2016). Volberg and colleagues (1999) compared gambling motivations in different ethnic groups and found that African Americans view gambling more as a means to win money, whereas Hispanics consider it more of a social activity. These motivational elements may partly explain the develop-ment of problems, as other research has identified financial motivations to be a key factor in the development of gambling problems (MacLaren et al. 2015; Clarke et al. 2006).

Comorbidity with ill-health and substance use problems

Substantial research shows that problem gambling co-occurs with mental health problems and substance use. Population and clinical studies demonstrate con-sistently that problem gambling is higher in populations with comorbid dis-orders, but causality cannot be attributed only to gambling. Most likely, common factors underlie both gambling and ill-health, and evidence is strong that they have reinforcing effects. Problem gambling and its comorbidities constitute a 'multi-morbid' (Kessler et al. 2008) negative health spiral in which the different disorders in combination increase the severity of the condition. Comorbidity is associated with slower recovery, higher severity of illness, increased rates of recurrence, and greater psychosocial disability, as well as delays in help seeking (Holdsworth et al. 2012; Ibanez et al. 2001). This makes problem gambling a heterogeneous condition, which should also be taken into account in treatment (Sharp et al. 2015; Suomi et al. 2014). A longitudinal study of problem gamblers showed that one year after quitting gambling, the prevalence of comorbid dis-orders had also decreased (Hodgins et al. 2005).

Three factors account for the reinforcing effects among the various co-morbidities. First, individuals with simultaneous disorders are likely to ignore or defy risks of different types of games. Petry (2003) found that gamblers who had the highest overall levels of comorbidities preferred lotteries, EGMs, or races. Sports bettors and card players had fewer psychiatric conditions. Secondly, the causality between gambling and comorbid disorders is complex. Gambling may cause or contribute to other disorders, and the other disorders may cause or contribute to gambling problems. The two sets of problems may also reflect another underlying disorder (Shaffer and Korn 2002), and comorbidities may evolve over time, mutually intensifying one another (Holdsworth et al. 2012). To further complicate matters, gambling and some psychiatric disorders may be independent of each other. Thirdly, the gambling environment and cultural context may contribute to the complexity and severity of the combined effects. Some mental health issues, such as stigma and shame, can be stronger for Asian than for European or American players (Sobrun-Maharaj et al. 2012). Gamblers who play at land-based venues report higher levels of psychological distress and treatment seeking than players in online environments (Blaszczynski et al. 2016; Hopley et al. 2011).

Mental and physical ill-health

The most frequently co-occurring mental health problems are mood disorders (depression), anxiety disorders, and personality disorders (Lorains et al. 2011; Petry et al. 2005; Haydock et al. 2015; Ladd and Petry 2003). Also, the incidence of suicide and other premature mortality is higher than average among those who experience gambling problems (Thon et al. 2014; Wong et al. 2010a; b; Jason et al. 1990). Table 5.2 provides a summary of these findings, based on a meta-analysis of population studies by Lorains and colleagues (2011).

Prevalence rates are much higher in clinical samples, estimated to be 80% for major depression in a systematic review (Delfabbro 2009). Elevated rates of dysthymic disorder, a chronic type of depression, are also linked to problem

Table 5.2 Prevalence of comorbid disorders in problem and pathological gamblers

Comorbid disorder	%
Major depression	23.1
Bipolar disorder/manic episodes	9.8
Any anxiety disorder	37.4
Generalized anxiety disorder	11.1
Any mood disorder	37.9
Antisocial personality disorder	28.8
Substance use disorders	57.5
Nicotine dependence	60.1

Reproduced from Lorains, F. K., Cowlishaw, S. and Thomas, S. A. (2011), Prevalence of comorbid disorders in problem and pathological gambling: systematic review and meta-analysis of population surveys. Addiction, 106: 490–498 with permission from Wiley.

gambling (Chou and Afifi 2011). Studies have suggested that family dysfunction or personality factors may explain both gambling problems and depression (Quigley et al. 2015; Miller et al. 2013), while others have suggested that emotionally vulnerable gamblers may seek escape from negative emotions and depression (Blaszczynski and Nower 2002; Wood and Griffiths 2007). In any case, depressive symptoms may exacerbate problem gambling and vice versa (Quigley et al. 2015; Thomsen et al. 2009), and depressive individuals may have more difficulty to quit gambling (Hodgins et al. 2005; Hodgins and el-Guebaly 2004).

Anxiety is another condition that has been commonly observed among problem gamblers (Chou and Afifi 2011; Bland et al. 1993). A large twin-study (Giddens et al. 2011) found that similar genetic and environmental factors contribute to both problem gambling and anxiety disorder. A similar explanation by third factors has been suggested for bipolar disorder, which has been connected to problem gambling in a number of clinical and population studies (Di Nicola et al. 2014; McIntyre et al. 2007; Kennedy et al. 2010). Di Nicola and co-workers (2014) note that comorbid bipolar and gambling disorder patients experience a more severe course of illness and poorer treatment outcome, due to a range of clinical and psychosocial factors that collectively impede recovery.

Attention deficit hyperactivity disorder (ADHD) is associated with gambling and problem gambling particularly among young males (Clark et al. 2013; Ariyabuddhiphongs 2013) and in adults with a history of childhood ADHD (Breyer et al. 2009; Carlton et al. 1987), although not all studies agree (Canu and Schatz 2011). Those with childhood ADHD symptoms that persist into adulthood have reported more severe gambling problems than those with non-persistent ADHD (Breyer et al. 2009). Studies among adult samples have identified ADHD in approximately 20% of problem gamblers (Chamberlain et al. 2015; Specker et al. 1995).

Obsessive-compulsive or impulse disorders (Bland et al. 1993; Odlaug et al. 2012; Durdle et al. 2008), schizophrenia (Desai and Potenza 2009; Black and Moyer 1998), avoidant, antisocial and paranoid personality disorders (Odlaug et al. 2012; Pietrzak and Petry 2005), as well as phobias and panic disorder (Chou and Afifi 2011) have been found to be associated with pathological gambling.

Gambling is also associated with a variety of physical health issues, including headaches, high blood pressure, cardiac arrest, arthritis, indigestion, weight loss, tachycardia, angina, cirrhosis, and Parkinson's disease (Chun et al. 2011; Morasco et al. 2006; Potenza et al. 2002; Santangelo et al. 2013). One comparative study (Black et al. 2013) found that the problem gambling group had more medical and mental health conditions, was more likely to avoid regular exercise, and had more emergency room visits and psychiatric admissions, compared with controls. The causality of these health consequences cannot be established, as gambling can both cause negative health outcomes and serve as a coping mechanism to escape physical or emotional problems (e.g., Parhami et al. 2014, Barry et al. 2013).

Substance use

Some characteristics of problem gamblers resemble those of heavy drinkers, frequent tobacco smokers, and illicit drug users. These characteristics include delay discounting and impulsivity (Audrain-McGovern et al. 2009; Reynolds 2006), suggesting possible common underlying mechanisms. Moreover, the diagnostic criteria for pathological gambling have been modeled on those of substance use disorders with respect to such features as tolerance (need to increase exposure to obtain same effects); unsuccessful attempts to quit; and jeopardizing important social, occupational or recreational activities. Such common characteristics, along with the professional framing of the disorders in parallel terms, may—at least in part—explain why we often see a substantial overlap between these addictive behaviors.

Substance use disorders are the most common conditions co-occurring with problem gambling (Petry et al. 2005). Sometimes called co-addiction (e.g., Fulton 2015) a majority of pathological gamblers suffer from substance use disorders (57%) (Table 5.2). Higher rates have been found in clinical samples. A meta-analysis of studies on patients seeking treatment for substance abuse found a weighed mean rate for problem gambling of 13.7% (Cowlishaw et al. 2014).

In addition to a syndrome-level association, pathological gambling and alcohol consumption co-occur at an event-level. In an interview study conducted among non-pathological gamblers, 80% reported consuming between four and ten drinks of alcohol while gambling on EGMs (Baron and Dickerson 1999). Drinking while gambling has been linked to higher severity of gambling problems (el-Guebaly et al. 2006), and problem gamblers are more likely to report being drunk or high while gambling compared to other gamblers (Martins et al. 2010). Gambling under the influence of alcohol results in larger bets and reduces the perception of consequences of risk taking (Shaffer and Korn 2002; see also Chapter 11).

Nicotine dependence is the most common comorbid condition among pathological gamblers not only at the syndrome level (Table 5.2), but also at the event level (McGrath and Barrett 2009; see also Chapter 11). A New Zealand study (Sullivan and Beer 2003) has shown that those with gambling problems increase their smoking when gambling. Like other forms of comorbidity, tobacco use and gambling may share common genetic social and environmental factors. The calming and stimulating effects of tobacco smoking may make gambling more pleasurable, and the stimulus of the game may prompt the desire to smoke (see Grant et al. 2009).

Problematic gambling, substance use, and ill-health co-occur, have mutual reinforcing effects, and resist positive change when they appear in combination. Compared to other problem gamblers, those with a comorbid substance use disorder gamble more often, have other psychiatric disorders, have more legal difficulties, and family problems, and are more likely to be unemployed (Petry et al. 2005). Comorbidities with substance use increase the complexity of providing treatment for problem gambling (Hodgins and el-Guebaly 2010).

As with mental illness, the causal sequencing of problem gambling and substance use remains uncertain. Some studies have suggested that substance use disorders predominantly predate problem gambling (French et al. 2008; Cunningham-Williams and Cottler 2001), but the reverse can also be true. A study in different US states showed that states that legalized gambling experienced a 5% increase in alcohol consumption (Sabbagh 2013). It is also possible that common factors, such as neurobiological processes or genetic and environmental contributions, may increase the risk for both conditions (Grant et al. 2002).

Although the links between gambling problems and substance use disorder have been demonstrated consistently, there have been significant variations in prevalence rates. This may be partly explained by sampling and differences in interview measures, but also by differences between cultural contexts and games. Results from non-western prevalence studies differ significantly from the averages described in Table 5.2. An Argentinian study (Abait and Folino 2007) found that 84% of pathological gamblers reported nicotine dependence while only 12.6% reported alcohol abuse. A South Korean survey showed that 47% of problem gamblers reported drug abuse (Lee 2002), while in a Singapore sample of pathological gamblers seeking treatment, only 7.3% reported substance abuse and 4.7% reported alcohol abuse (Teo et al. 2007).

Suicide and premature mortality

Problem and pathological gamblers have elevated rates of suicidal thoughts, suicide attempts, and completed suicides (e.g., Moghaddam et al. 2015; Thon et al. 2014; Wong et al. 2014; Wong et al. 2010a; b; Newman 2007; Wynne 2002). Suicidal intentions and suicide may be linked to gambling by way of excessive debts and escalation of problems, or they can be a part of comorbid depression, ensuing relationship problems or humiliation (Fulton 2015), although there have also been contesting views, mainly from the industry side (Thon et al. 2014).

It is difficult to estimate the exact role of gambling in completed suicides in epidemiological studies (McCleary et al. 2002; Shaffer and Korn 2002), but a growing body of evidence links suicides directly to gambling. Ecological studies reinforce the view that gambling and suicide are linked. Las Vegas has the highest suicide rate in the United States (Phillips et al. 1997) both for residents and for visitors. Wray et al. (2008) have shown that the odds of suicide are 50% greater among Las Vegas residents than among residents elsewhere, and visitors to Las Vegas doubled their risk for suicide compared to those who stayed in their home county or visited another destination. Leaving Las Vegas was associated with a 20% reduction in risk for suicide. High suicide levels have also been found in Atlantic City after casinos were opened (Phillips et al. 1997).

Conclusion

The epidemiological and clinical research reviewed in this chapter indicates that the prevalence of (problem) gambling varies with age, gender, ethnic background, and socio-economic status. Problem gambling relative to overall participation rates is more prevalent in younger age groups compared to middle aged and older persons. Problem gambling rates are often found to be higher—although overall participation rates are lower than average—in lower socio-economic groups, the unemployed, and persons on welfare. Gambling problems occur frequently among populations that are already vulnerable for other reasons, particularly for substance use and mental health issues. There is evidence that gambling is a causal factor in suicides at the population level. But it remains an open question how much problem gambling causes co-occurring problems and socio-economic deprivation, or how much it is the consequence of these. Nevertheless, government officials, regulators, and policymakers have to face the fundamental ethical question: To what extent is the financial exploitation of already troubled and marginalized populations through policies that facilitate gambling consistent with considerations of social justice?

While these covariations have been affirmed, methodological problems in measuring problem rates and gambling prevalence cause uncertainties in tracking trends and comparing populations. Trends derived from population surveys will be subject to weaknesses of survey methods and other sources of error. Findings based on diagnostic problem gambling scores are less useful than concrete measures of harm for understanding gambling as a reinforcing factor in difficult life situations. Given the current state of gambling epidemiology, the best policy outcome measures are (1) various measures of harm to others and to the gambler, and (2) the two total consumption measures (total wager and GGR) from official or industry statistics that were used in Chapter 3.

Sometimes these are available according to gambling mode, which is very useful from a policy perspective. Although such global measures do not directly inform the estimation of problem prevalence, relevant inferences can be made from them, as implied by the Total Consumption Model to be discussed in the next chapter.

Three conclusions can be derived from population surveys on gambling prevalence. First, the number of people who participate in some form of gambling activity at least once a year is quite high in many countries. Gambling is not an exclusive activity that only very few people engage in, especially in countries where it is legal, accessible, and commercialized. Second, only a small fraction of the population shows evidence of problem gambling at any one time, while the number of people affected is much larger because each gambler causes harm to many others and there is great fluidity of individuals among the problem gamblers, meaning that their number over time is much larger than cross-sectional surveys suggest. The third conclusion returns us to the issue of social justice: survey research conducted in many countries indicates that gambling problems tend to be concentrated, though not exclusively, in the most vulnerable and disadvantaged groups, including ethnic minorities, the homeless, the unemployed, the mentally ill, alcohol and drug users, and those who have lower incomes and socio-economic status. Gambling transfers wealth from the most frequent gamblers to owners of the operating companies, to the government authorities, and to the beneficiaries of direct contributions to "good causes".

Chapter 6

The total volume of gambling and the prevalence of gambling problems

One of the leading paradigms in public health epidemiology focuses on the relationship between heavy use involving elevated risk and the degree of participation in the behavior by general populations including moderate users and sometimes even abstainers. It has been observed that the number of heavy users and also their level of risk is higher in populations with high total consumption by those who use at all. In other words, the number and consumption level of heavy users corresponds to average (per user) consumption, being low in populations with low total consumption and higher in populations with a higher average population level. This applies both across populations and within the same population when its average level changes. The approach based on these observations is called the *total consumption model* (TCM). It has been influential in the arguments underlying alcohol policymaking, because it implies that to reduce the amount of risk due to heavy use, the consumption of those whose consumption level is low or moderate is also a relevant consideration. Intuitively, one would think that the TCM fits the gambling area. This chapter evaluates to what extent this model applies to gambling and gambling problems on the basis of its theoretical assumptions and empirical evidence.

The skewed distribution of gambling behavior

A key factor determining incidence and prevalence is how the population is distributed in different groups by the intensity of play. The distribution of gambling frequency or gambling expenditures refers to the proportions of the population that are involved in gambling along a continuum ranging from zero (no gambling, no expenditures) to the highest level (frequent gambling, high expenditures). If gambling followed a *normal distribution* among gamblers, there would be few infrequent gamblers and few excessive gamblers, with the greatest proportion of the population clustering around some average or central value. Typically this is not the case in most activities in which individuals engage with variable intensity. Figure 6.1 illustrates a very common

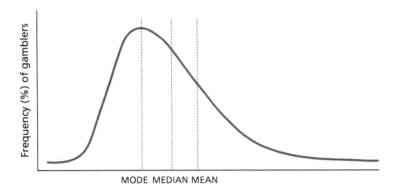

Gambling behavior (e.g. gambling frequency, gambling expenditures)

Fig 6.1 Illustrative curve demonstrating a unimodal distribution skewed to the right, as applied to gambling

statistical pattern in which most individuals in a population are either not users at all or use very little, whereas a small number of them account for a very large share of total use. Such distributions are called *unimodal* as they have only one peak (*mode*) and they are *skewed to the right*, which means that most people (non-users and moderate users) are clustered at the lower end of the continuum whereas the heaviest users are distributed along a long tail at the right. The *median* level, or the point that divides the population into two equal halves, is lower than the average (*mean*), because heavy users weigh heavily in the average, pushing it to the right. The unimodal and continuous nature of the curve implies that the "heaviest" gamblers are not a separate population, distinct from other gamblers in terms of how often they gamble or how much they spend on gambling, irrespective of any cut-off value or criteria for problem gambling. Moreover, it implies that a small fraction of gamblers account for a very large fraction of all gambling activities and of all gambling expenditures, as demonstrated by Chipman et al. (2006), Williams and Wood (2004), and Livingstone and Woolley (2007). The same kind of unimodal asymmetrical distribution has been observed for alcohol consumption (Skog 1985; Rossow and Clausen 2013) and many other behaviors and population characteristics.

The total consumption model

The relationship between total alcohol consumption (or mean per capita consumption) and prevalence of excessive drinking was first noted by the French demographer Sully Ledermann (1956), who found a strong regularity in the distribution of alcohol consumption in different populations with very different mean consumption levels. The Norwegian alcohol researcher Ole-Jørgen Skog

(1985) took Ledermann's work further. He offered a theory of the collectivity of drinking practices by which drinkers at different levels of quantity and frequency move up and down together due to social interaction and interdependency. This implies that an increase in average consumption in a population is accompanied, not only by an increase in the prevalence of excessive drinkers, but by an increase in *consumption at all consumption levels*—and *vice versa*.

Given the strong association between heavy use and risk of alcohol-related harm, we should also expect an association between total consumption and rate of harm (see Figure 6.2). This is indeed reported in numerous studies both across populations and within populations for alcohol-related problems such as liver cirrhosis, violence, homicide, and suicide (Babor et al. 2010; Norström and Ramstedt 2005), although exceptions to this have also been noted (see for instance Meier 2010).

The total consumption model is applied and interpreted in two slightly different ways. Some authors have referred to the model as the single distribution theory, thereby addressing only the relationship between total consumption and the prevalence of heavy drinkers (or excessive users) (Rossow and Norström 2013; Raninen et al. 2014). Other authors have emphasized that the total consumption of alcohol determines the amount of alcohol-related problems in a population (Sulkunen and Warsell 2012). The latter relationship is not obvious, as many alcohol-related harms including health problems can occur also at low consumption levels (Edwards et al. 1994). Nevertheless, there is strong empirical support for both views: total consumption of alcohol is associated with the prevalence of heavy drinkers and the rate of alcohol-related harm.

The total consumption model is also supported in other health-related areas. A strong association between population mean and prevalence of high risk individuals has been reported for hypertension from 52 population samples from 31 countries (Rose and Day 1990). Its prevalence was closely related to mean blood pressure; that is, the higher the mean blood pressure in a population the higher the prevalence of hypertension. Correspondingly, prevalence of obesity was associated with mean body mass index, and excessive intake of sodium was associated with mean sodium consumption. Based on these observations, Rose

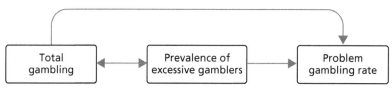

Fig 6.2 Assumed associations between total consumption, prevalence of excessive users, and harm rate in a population

and Day (1990 p.1033) conclude—much in line with Skog's (1985) notion—that "the distribution of each of these variables moves up or down as a coherent whole: the tail belongs to the body, and the deviants are a part of the population."

The validity of the total consumption model with respect to gambling

Gambling and alcohol consumption share a number of relevant characteristics within a public health perspective. In both behaviors, the risk of many problems increases steeply with the intensity (frequency and quantity) of the behavior. Like alcohol use, gambling is widely practiced in many societies. Problem gamblers gamble more frequently, place higher bets, and spend more money on gambling than other gamblers (Rossow and Molde 2006; Currie et al. 2006; Livingstone and Woolley 2007; Orford et al. 2013). Therefore, if changes in the total amount of gambling in a society are accompanied by similar changes in the tail of the distribution, as is the case for alcohol use, an increase in total amount of gambling is also expected to be accompanied by an increase in problem gambling (as illustrated in Figure 6.2).

As in alcohol studies, the total consumption model has been applied in two ways in gambling research. Some studies have addressed the relationship between total amount of gambling and heavy (or excessive) use (e.g., Lund 2008; Grun and McKeigue 2000). Other studies have addressed total gambling and prevalence of problem gambling (e.g., Markham et al. 2014). Still other studies have adopted both approaches (Govoni 2000; Hansen and Rossow 2008). For the sake of simplicity, we will here use the term total consumption model (TCM) for both of these associations.

With respect to gambling, the terms "consumption" and "heavy or excessive use" need to be operationalized. Possible measures for total amount of gambling in a society include gambling expenditures (total wager) and total losses by gamblers (gross gambling revenue GGR for operators) per year. Alternatively, surveys measure gambling frequency (e.g., number of times gambled per year) and individual spending that can be aggregated over the total population and specific sub-populations. Excessive and problem gambling can be operationalized in several ways as well: 1) gambling expenditures above a fixed value; 2) expenditures above a proportion of income; 3) total gambling frequency above a fixed value (e.g., > 300 times per year), or 4) using various diagnostic instruments (e.g., SOGS, NODS, DSM-5 or PGSI).

Four issues should be kept in mind when applying a model derived from alcohol consumption to gambling. First, the TCM for alcohol is concerned with the consumption distribution among drinkers. Changes in the proportion of current drinkers are common, but the TCM does not speak to this, and there is no clear model in the literature for this relationship. The percentages of people who have gambled in the last year are typically lower than the percentages for drinking in the last year. In high-income countries, the latter range from about 75% to 95% (World Health Organization 2014), whereas for gambling the percentages range from about 50% to 80% (Williams et al. 2012a).

Second, the TCM for alcohol does not distinguish between different alcoholic beverages. There are substantial cultural differentiations between alcoholic beverages in terms of contexts of use and who drinks them, but alcohol use in whatever form and way has similar social and health effects. In contrast, gambling is highly variable in its forms, effects, and consequences. There are large differences between types of gambling in terms of the risk of excessive gambling and harm. The relationship between frequency of play and problem gambling is particularly pronounced for EGMs (and VLTs), and internet and sports gambling have the highest conversion rates from having tried the activity to frequent play (Holtgraves 2009a). The substantial variations between the modes and patterns of gambling may mean that they should not be treated as a single class of behavior in TCM analyzes.

Third, TCM studies have usually treated national populations as single entities, but differences between males and females, regions, religious, and ethnic groups may be so significant that the theory might not work across such social divides (Skog 2001). The two clusters of gamblers found by Holtgraves (2009a) among Canadians suggest that national populations may not fit a single model in TCM analyses. In many studies participation in national lotteries is treated separately from other forms of gambling for a similar reason.

Fourth, the distributions may be different for alcohol use and for gambling. There is little question that the distribution of gambling behavior is skewed to the right, so that a high proportion of gambling (and gambling losses) is attributable to a small fraction of all gamblers. But the exact form of the distribution may differ from the lognormal or gamma distributions commonly found for alcohol (Rehm et al. 2010). There is an upper limit on a particular person's consumption of alcohol in a given period of time, while in many circumstances there is no effective limit on the amount which a single human can gamble. This means that the concentration of gambling expenditures can be even higher than in alcohol consumption.

With these reservations in mind, the relationship between average consumption and heavy or problematic use holds for most types of gambling as well as for aggregated participation in populations so far studied. Richard Govoni (2000) was among the first to apply the theory to gambling. Data from three cross-sectional surveys in the adult population of the city of Windsor in Ontario,

Canada, showed that gambling expenditures followed a skewed lognormal distribution with a long right tail. Moreover, a straight linear association between mean gambling expenditures and prevalence of excessive gambling was observed. A strong positive association was found between mean expenditures and the proportion of households spending above 15% of family income on gambling. A strong association between gambling expenditures and prevalence of pathological gambling (SOGS score 5+) was also found.

Another early study, Grun and McKeigue (2000), used data from two cross-sectional surveys collected before and after the introduction of a national lottery in the United Kingdom. The distribution of gambling expenditures was found to be skewed and the percentage of those spending above 20 GBP per week and of those spending more than 10% of household income was positively associated with mean as well as median expenditure in the population. Average gambling expenditures more than doubled after introduction of the lottery. The cumulative frequency distributions for the two survey years showed that the increase in mean expenditures was accompanied by a rightward shift of the entire distribution, including the right tail—the top few percentiles. The proportion of those who had gambled at all almost doubled, whereas the prevalence of excessive gambling increased by a factor of at least three.

Three studies from Norway give support to the TCM. Lund (2008) analyzed data from three population surveys (two adult samples and one adolescent sample) and found that the distribution of gambling frequency resembled a lognormal distribution, and was thus unimodal and skewed to the right. Some 11% to 15% of those who had gambled exceeded twice the mean gambling frequency. Comparisons of sub-samples with different means showed that groups with a higher mean gambling frequency (e.g., males) were characterized by more gambling along the whole gambling frequency continuum than groups with a lower mean gambling frequency (e.g., females). A clear positive relationship between mean gambling frequency and the proportion of frequent gamblers was established in all three data sets.

Another Norwegian study (Hansen and Rossow 2008) analyzed data from several school surveys of teenagers. The distributions of gambling frequency and gambling expenditures were skewed to the right. Some 11% to 13% gambled more than twice as often as the average and the 10% who had gambled most frequently accounted for half of all gambling occasions and total expenditures in the sample. Teenagers meeting DSM criteria for problem gambling accounted for a disproportionately large fraction of all gambling occasions and gambling expenditures. Strong positive associations were observed between excessive gambling (frequent gambling, high expenditures, or problem gambling) and indicators of total gambling (mean gambling frequency and mean gambling expenditures) in the samples. While the two Norwegian studies from 2008 compared cross-sectional sub-samples, Hansen and Rossow (2012) also studied a change in total gambling (mean gambling frequency) from one year to another. They found that the significant *decrease* in mean gambling frequency that occurred in Norway from 2005 to 2006 was indeed accompanied by a *decrease* in gambling frequency at all levels of gambling: light, moderate, frequent, and excessive gamblers all decreased their gambling frequency when examined at group levels.

Using data from Australia and New Zealand, Abbott (2006) showed a positive relationship between EGM expenditures and prevalence of problem gambling. An exceptionally powerful Australian study (Markham et al. 2014) tested the TCM by combining problem gambling data from a large household survey with information about gambling expenditures on electronic gaming machines (EGMs) at the venue level. The study established that prevalence of problem gambling correlated significantly with monthly EGM expenditures per adult ($r = 0.27$). Furthermore, the prevalence of problem gamblers doubled (from 9% to 18%) with an increase in mean monthly EGM expenditures from 10 to 150 AUD per adult. Within this range, each increase in expenditure by 20 AUD was associated with an estimated average 1.7 percentage point increase in the proportion of problem gamblers (Markham et al. 2014).

Table 6.1 summarizes the studies that address the validity of the TCM in gambling.

The term excessive gambling is used to cover both frequent gambling and high gambling expenditures, each defined in slightly different ways in the different studies.

Ideally, research needs to examine how changes in total gambling relate to the prevalence of excessive gambling and problem gambling. Unfortunately, there have been few attempts to analyze changes in problem prevalence in relation to total gambling within a single jurisdiction, such as the studies by Grun and McKeigue (2000) and Hansen and Rossow (2012). An alternative approach is to correlate spatial variation in total gambling and prevalence of problem gambling. For this book we obtained and summarized data on prevalence of problem gambling, pathological gambling, and gambling expenditures as percentages of household budget from 12 European countries (Austria, Belgium, Denmark, Finland, France, Germany, Hungary, Italy, Netherlands, Norway, Sweden, and the United Kingdom). A moderate positive correlation between prevalence of problem gambling and gambling expenditures was observed (bi-variate $r = 0.28$) which was only slightly modified by adjusting for the relative importance of more problem prone games (casinos and EGMs) ($r = 0.37$).

Table 6.1 Overview of studies addressing the total consumption model with respect to gambling

	Non-gamblers included in analyzes	Cross-sectional or longitudinal comparison	Association of total gambling and prevalence of excessive gambling	Association of total gambling and prevalence of problem gambling
Govoni 2000	No	Cross-sectional	Mean expenditures - % spending > 3000 CAD (adj $R^2 = .66$) Mean expenditures - % > 15% family income (adj $R^2 = .80$)	Mean expenditures - % SOGS score 5+ (adj $R^2 = .83$)
Grun and McKeigue 2000	Yes	Both	Mean expenditures - % > 20 GBP/ week (regr coeff 1.6) Mean expenditures - % > 10% household income (regr coeff 1.2)	
Lund 2008	Yes	Cross-sectional	Mean gambling frequency - % frequent gamblers (clear positive relationship, not quantified)	
Hansen and Rossow 2008	Yes	Cross-sectional	Mean expenditures on EGMs - % high expenditures ($r = .73$, $r = .57$) Mean gambling frequency - % weekly gamblers ($r = .90$; $r = .83$)	Mean expenditures on EGMs - % LieBet score 2 ($r = .63$; $r = .60$) Mean gambling frequency - % meeting various DSM-criteria ($r = .52$; $r = .47$; $r = .33$)
Hansen and Rossow 2012	No	Longitudinal	Mean gambling frequency – percentiles of gambling frequency (50th, 75th, 90th, 95th): clear positive relationship, not quantified	

Table 6.1 Continued

	Non-gamblers included in analyzes	Cross-sectional or longitudinal comparison	Association of total gambling and prevalence of excessive gambling	Association of total gambling and prevalence of problem gambling
Abbott 2006	Not clear	Cross-sectional		Mean EGM expenditures - % SOGS 5+: positive relationship, not quantified
Markham et al. 2014	No	Cross-sectional		Mean expenditures on EGMs - % PGSI 2+ (r = .27)

Risk curves

The TCM approach, which looks at the relationship between the total (or per capita) amount of gambling and the harm caused by it (rather than heavy use) in a population, needs to account for how the probability of each type of harm is related to the consumption level. For alcohol-related harms, there are three main types of risk curves. For accidents, the probability increases steadily with the amount of use: even moderate levels of intoxication elevate the probability of falls and other accidents (Taylor et al. 2010). For ischemic heart disease, a wide research literature exists on the possibility that, compared to abstention, modest use of alcohol actually decreases the risk of disease, whereas high consumption increases the risk (Roerecke and Rehm 2014). This is called the J-shaped curve. Finally, other problems, like liver cirrhosis, are mostly related to quite heavy use, resembling an exponential risk curve. In policy terms, the latter type of risk curve could imply that prevention strategies should aim at the small fraction of very heavy users, rather than the total population.

A similar argument has been proposed in research on gambling. The responsible gambling policy promoted by the gambling industry rests on the notion that there is no risk at low levels of participation or of player losses; in other words, problems start to occur only after a certain threshold of spending. One study found low-risk thresholds at a level as high as 500–1000 Canadian dollars per year (Currie et al. 2006). Another study (Currie et al. 2008) found this level to span from 138 to about 1000 Canadian dollars per year, and a study in the United States identified the risk threshold at 1.9% of monthly income (Weinstock et al. 2007). If generalized, these results imply that policies could aim to keep individual player loss levels down and accept that the total consumption could stay the same or even increase if reduction of heavy use could be compensated for by an increase of play at the level with no or only an acceptable risk involved. An exponential risk curve would imply further that the harm level strongly depends on the intensity of play (frequency and volume) among those who gamble. If the total (per capita) consumption increased because new moderate players are recruited from among those who do not gamble, the level of harm would not be expected to increase much. On the other hand, if the total consumption increases because those who do gamble intensify their participation, the problem level will soar with the rising average. Based on such assumptions, a policy attempting to suppress problems caused by heavy gambling would be directed at reducing the number of intensive players among the gambling population, by changing the consumption curve to reduce its skewness. Unless new players would be recruited to the low end of the consumption distribution, the total volume of gambling would decline. The success of such a policy strongly depends on the risk curves, and according to the TCM the outcome is unlikely except in cases where the whole gambling mix changes from intensive to less intensive games.

A secondary analysis of data from four countries (Australia, Finland, Canada, and Norway) found no evidence to support the J-curve hypothesis known from alcohol studies. Instead, the risk curves for problem gambling indicators were r-shaped for total gambling losses as well as for most game types, with a rapidly increasing risk at initial loss levels reaching a plateau as the loss levels increase. Losses in EGM use drive the risk level up faster than most other games, whereas linear risk curves were found for racing, lotteries, and sports betting in some countries (Markham et al. 2016). A Finnish study (Raisamo et al. 2015a) supports this result, examining both gambling frequency and player losses (spending minus wins) as exposure variables. Both were related to harm even at low levels, also controlling for demographic factors. Thus, these studies suggest that overall harm level in society should be expected to rise in a fairly linear fashion with rising volumes and frequencies of gambling.

However, research on the consumption distribution as well as on the risk curves is uncommon in the gambling area, and the relationships between total per capita gambling (in terms of spending on games or gambling frequency), level of experienced and reported harm, and the types of games played are not conclusive. In any case, the stability of the consumption curve in combination with the likely shapes of various risk curves, points to the conclusion that increases in total gambling volumes lead to increases in harms. If the risk curves are linear, or even exponential, harm levels are very sensitive to heavy gambling in populations where the average level is high. These are likely to be very serious types of problems in society. In contrast, r-shaped curves imply that small increases in gambling activities will lead to rising problems even at moderate gambling levels; perhaps the problems will be less severe but affect larger numbers of people (Browne et al. 2016). Why the increase in some risks should slow down with increasing intensity of play is a question that gambling research cannot answer for the moment. Many factors might contribute to explaining this finding, including methodological issues and the possibility that many heavy gamblers may stop after their losses have exhausted their resources or brought their behavior to the attention of their families, friends or other affected persons.

Availability theory and adaptation theory

Closely related to the total consumption model is *availability theory*. This is the assumption that changes in the availability of gambling opportunities will have effects on total amount of activity, and consequently on the total quantity of related harm as predicted by the TCM (Lund 2008; Welte et al. 2007). The possible impact of availability on gambling and on gambling problems will be addressed in Chapter 7; here results from some correlational studies on EGM availability and problem gambling are summarized.

Cross-sectional correlations between EGM availability (EGMs per 1000 persons) and problem gambling prevalence within countries have in some analyses been found to be positive and fairly large. Among eight Australian states/territories in 1999 the correlation with SOGS 5+ prevalence was highly significant ($r = 0.74$, $p <.05$; our calculations based on Williams et al. 2012a, Table 3, p. 31). Abbott (2006) presented a scatter plot of EGM expenditures and prevalence of scoring 5+ on SOGS in nine jurisdictions in Australia and New Zealand in 1998, indicating a positive association. Attempting to quantify this association, we extracted data by visual inspection of the scatter plot in Abbott's paper (Abbott (2006) Figure 2, p. 15), which yielded a correlation coefficient of 0.78 ($p < .05$, our calculation). Correspondingly, Storer et al. (2009) analyzed problem gambling rates from 34 surveys in Australia and New Zealand since 1991 and found a positive correlation between problem gambling prevalence and EGM density. In the state of Victoria, Australia, Barratt and colleagues (2014) found a strong correlation between EGM density and measures of help-seeking for gambling problems, with a range of local factors controlled. Among ten Canadian provinces in 2002 the correlation was also strong ($r = 0.66$, $p <.05$) (Williams et al. 2012a). Thus, these associations are compatible with availability theory predictions.

However, across many and diverse countries (n = 54), the association is small, negative and statistically insignificant ($r = -0.26$, $p >.05$), our calculations based on Williams and colleagues (2012a, Table 4, p. 33). They explain the cross-country result by observing that in Asian countries, problem gambling rates are high but EGM densities are low, while in European countries, problem gambling rates are low whereas EGM densities are high, but with much lower bet and win sizes compared to other countries.

The association between gambling exposure and prevalence of problem gambling has also been challenged in some studies. In the Australian state of Victoria, recent data indicate that the use of EGMs and participation in most other gambling forms declined between 2003 and 2014. During this period, the number of EGMs remained constant but strong population growth reduced relative availability. As availability and average use of EGMs declined, availability theory would predict that also problem gambling should be reduced, but actually rates of problem gambling and moderate risk gambling (i.e., PGSI 3+ scores) remained constant. Gamblers in the PGSI 3+ group used EGMs more frequently in 2014 than in 2008. Average per capita expenditure among those who used EGMs increased in real terms from AUD 2,452 in 2003 to AUD 3,688 in 2014 (2014–15 values) (Hare 2015).

In this example, those who use EGMs were fewer but were more likely to be spending more money doing so in 2014 than in 2003 or 2008. Prevalence evidence suggests they also were at greater risk of experiencing harm than in 2003 or 2008.

An alternative approach to availability theory, known as *adaptation theory* (Shaffer et al. 1997; Shaffer 2005; Abbott 2006), suggests that exposure to new forms of gambling (particularly EGMs and other high-intensity games) increases problems, but over time 'host immunity' and protective environmental changes lead to reduced problem levels, even in the face of increasing gambling accessibility and exposure. It is assumed that over time, people will adapt and become more able to counter gambling problems, and consequently problem prevalence is likely to fall (Abbott 2006).

Empirical findings have been offered to support this approach. Welte and colleagues (2002) found that among seven regions in the United States, New England had the highest mean gambling frequency but also the lowest rate of problem gambling. It should be noted that the prevalence figures in this study are based on very small numbers; the total sample in New England comprised 139 respondents and only three or four problem gamblers. Norwegian data from two population surveys showed a very modest increase in pathological gambling (from 0.15% in 1997 to 0.3% in 2002) in a period of increasing EGM gambling. Again, the very low prevalence figures (the numbers of pathological gamblers in the 1997 and 2002 surveys were 3 and 16, respectively) limit assessment of real changes (Lund and Nordlund 2003). Different measurement instruments and response rates in the two surveys also hamper comparability.

Abbott and colleagues (2016) conclude that neither simple availability nor simple adaptation theory is supported. In their Victorian study, for example, they report a significant increase in young adult problem prevalence despite a large decrease in weekly gambling participation by the whole population. Similar results have been obtained in Sweden (Abbott et al. 2014) and Britain (Wardle et al. 2011a). In heterogeneous societies some sub-populations have experienced long-term exposure and show signs of adaptation, while other population sectors have been recently exposed. In these latter groups relatively low proportions of people participate, but those who do are exposed to a very high risk. They include youth, young adults, and recent migrants from societies with lower exposure to gambling (Abbott et al. 2016).

One of the criticisms that can be levelled at adaptation theory is that it leaves unclear why adaptation might occur. Williams et al. (2012a) suggested that people might gradually become aware of the potential harms of the new game or of gambling generally. Participation might decrease after the novelty has worn off, and industry and government might increase their efforts to provide gambling more safely.

On the other hand, many confounding factors, in addition to measurement problems, may make adaptation a spurious interpretation of the statistical observations. Methodological issues plague prevalence studies and may render them unreliable. Simultaneous changes in the composition of the population (age structure, immigration, educational level) and the relative availability of game types should be controlled for; game mix might have changed; unregistered participation, and the ecology of game placement might make the population appear to "adapt". The incidence of new cases of problem gambling might even go down because those most at risk have been effectively removed from the pool of people with gambling problems due to severe consequences such as bankruptcy or suicide. Finally, saturation of the market may play a role. New games usually add volume to the overall gambling activity but at high levels of participation they also substitute for older games (Marionneau and Nikkinen 2017).

Adaptation theory might be relevant for an understanding of the global increase in gambling expenditures (GGR) and the parallel decrease in problem gambling rates in recent years. The methodological difficulties discussed already also apply at this level. First, prevalence figures from surveys in various countries and over time are not directly comparable. Different data collection methods, sampling procedures, non-response rates, and very low problem prevalence may limit conclusions that can be drawn from data. Moreover, as high-intensity games have steeper risk curves and therefore are more likely to cause problem gambling than others, redistribution of GGR in their favor is more relevant than expenditures across all games. Further, concentration of availability in areas where utilization and expenditures may be higher than population averages may distort the pattern. As Markham and Young (2015) demonstrate, and Abbott et al. (2016) concede, the geographical location of EGMs has been adjusted by the industry to maximize revenue.

As a general rule, population levels of gambling tend to go up and down with availability, and gambling problems can be expected to follow these variations. However, the examples discussed in the previous paragraph demonstrate that population level effects and the total volume or frequency of participation that cause them may not be sufficient considerations. Game types and gambling environments as well as differential degrees of vulnerability among population sub-groups must be taken into account in policymaking. In some cases no change in problem gambling prevalence with increasing or decreasing availability may indicate that part of the population has adapted its behavior, others have been recruited as new users, and some vulnerable groups may be experiencing reduced resources to gamble.

Conclusion and policy implications

Research on the distribution of gambling behavior is still sparse. The findings in the few studies addressing this issue are nevertheless fairly consistent. They demonstrate a skew distribution of gambling, which implies that a small fraction of gamblers account for a very large fraction of all gambling activities and of all gambling expenditures. This distribution also implies that, irrespective of cut-off values or criteria for problem gambling, the "heaviest" gamblers are not distinctly separate from other gamblers. Studies demonstrate a clear link between the mean gambling level and prevalence of excessive (or heavy) and problem gambling in a population. These findings correspond well to those consistently found with respect to alcohol consumption.

The study of the average is crucial for understanding the dynamics of social change and interactions (possibly reciprocal) between the majority and those whose behavior is the most extreme. The problems of heavy users, always a minority of any population, cannot be separated from the behavior of the majority.

The total consumption model has direct implications for policy. It suggests that the way most people gamble affects those who end up with problems. Consequently, strategies that effectively reduce gambling at the population level will likely also reduce problem gambling and related harms. But it also implies the reverse. As a disproportionately large fraction of gambling revenues stem from a very small proportion of problem gamblers, any successful effort to reduce their participation is likely to reduce the total volume of the trade, both directly and through interactional effects on moderate gamblers.

Availability of gambling opportunities, the total volume and frequency of the activity, and its effects on problem gambling prevalence in the whole population, are not the only considerations to be taken into account in policymaking that aims to promote the public interest. Also types of games, gambling environments, and the distribution of the burden among vulnerable and less vulnerable groups must be examined in assessments of policy alternatives.

Chapter 7

The effects of changing availability

We showed in Chapters 3 and 4 that the global growth of gambling activity has not occurred independently of government policies. Regulations have been relaxed, gambling opportunities have been expanded, and gambling participation and expenditures have risen. Technology, notably the internet and mobile phones have increased the availability of gambling dramatically in more recent years. Despite this historical development, the connection between availability, behavior, and gambling problems remains disputed.

Standard economic theory postulates that people make rational choices optimizing utility. An increase in the price and a reduction in physical availability increases "costs" to obtain the goods or services and therefore reduces demand. Availability in this broad sense refers to the ease of access to a commodity or a service including the effort required in terms of distance, sales hours, and other factors that add to the cost of purchase. Availability is also influenced by age limits and other restrictions on who is eligible to purchase or participate, limits on quantities or rations, and other constraints on the transactions between the market provider and the customer. All of these factors can, at least in theory, be regulated by public policy. However, as discussed below, price as a policy lever presents a special problem in the gambling market.

Social and cultural availability refers to the acceptance of gambling and the extent to which it is sanctioned by cultural norms or forbidden by religious injunctions, as in Islamic societies, but also to the attractiveness of a gambling venue. Moore et al. (2011) have distinguished between *social accessibility*, related to enjoying a gambling venue because it is a social place, and *accessible retreat*, which refers to venues that provide a geo-temporally available retreat from social interaction. Cognitive availability refers to knowledge or understanding about gambling.

This chapter considers the evidence on how policy changes have increased and—in far fewer cases—reduced the availability of gambling and how they have influenced behavior and related problems in different countries. The focus here is on availability at the population level, looking at the public's general exposure to gambling.

Physical availability

There is solid empirical evidence that availability of alcohol and tobacco influences the consumption of these substances as well as the prevalence of heavy use, dependence, and substance-related harm (Babor et al. 2010). Correspondingly, we may—*a priori*—expect that increases in availability will lead to increasing gambling behavior and gambling problems, and reductions in availability will reduce them. However, this is a *ceteris paribus* proposition—change in other factors in the situation may affect the outcomes, so that decreases in gambling and/or gambling problems may occur in the absence of availability restrictions, or the effect of availability changes may be countered by changes in other factors in the situation. Harm to society is a multidimensional consequence of the activity. Causal evidence on the impact of availability measures on behavioral variables is just a part of the picture, although an important one. Tables 7.1 and 7.2 summarize the results of studies of increased and reduced gambling availability, respectively. These studies are discussed in more detail in the remainder of the chapter.

Measuring the physical availability of gambling is a challenge. Studies have either measured distance to the closest gambling opportunity or the number of gambling operations in an area. Both are problematic. There can be many gambling opportunities at one spot, like a casino with many gambling machines and game tables, or gambling possibilities may be spread more equally throughout a city (Australian Productivity Commission 1999). Research has also shown that users visit most frequently the nearest gambling venue (Young et al. 2012). The farther people have to travel and the greater the effort required, the less people tend to gamble. Also, the higher the density of gambling in one area or the shorter the distance to the nearest venue, the more acceptable the gambling will appear, and the higher the participation (St-Pierre et al. 2014).

The relative rather than absolute strength or extent of availability regulations is important when evaluating their effects. For example, a new casino in a community where gambling is already widely available is less likely to have an impact as compared to a community with little or no access to gambling. The density and proximity of gambling opportunities interact with game types and the socio-economic structure of the population (Williams et al. 2011b). Continuous games (electronic gambling machines (EGMs) and online casino games) are considered especially harmful, and availability changes in these are more likely to have greater effects than other types of games.

Table 7.1 Studies of the impact of increased availability according to country, type of change, and outcomes.

Country	Availability Change	Year	Outcomes	References	Observations
AUSTRALIA	General increase in gambling availability	2003–2012	No increase in problem gambling; gambling participation declined	Abbott et al. 2016	Points towards adaptation model
AUSTRALIA	Permission to set up EGMs in hotels in Queensland	1991	Problem gambling increased	The Australian Institute of Gambling Research 1995	Also found positive effects on employment
CANADA	Opening of the gaming hall "Trois-Rivières" in Quebec	2007	No elevation in crime or increase in problem gambling	Alain 2011	
CANADA	Opening of "Hull" casino	1996	No increase in problem gambling rate	Jaques and Ladouceur 2006	
CANADA	Opening of "Niagara Falls" casino	1996	Gambling problems higher a year after opening the casino	Room et al. 1999	
CANADA	Opening of "Windsor" casino	1994	No increase in problem gambling rate; though higher demand for problem gambling counselling	Govoni et al. 1998	
FRANCE	Permitting licensed Internet gambling	2010	Increased participation, but decreased problem gambling, when compared to unregulated sites	Costes et al. 2015	

(continued)

Table 7.1 Continued

Country	Availability Change	Year	Outcomes	References	Observations
SWEDEN	Opening of two casinos	2001	Increased gambling problems in community of one of the casinos	Westfelt 2006	
SWITZERLAND	Permission to open 19 casinos	2002	No change in problem gambling	Bondolfi et al. 2008	Same time as prohibition of non-casino gambling machines and strict preventive measures inside casinos
UK	Introduction of the National Lottery	Mid-1990s	Excessive gambling increased	Grun and McKeigue 2000	
US	Opening of casinos in Kentucky	1993	No effect on bankruptcies	Boardman and Perry 2007	
US	Parishes allowed to set up EGMs in Louisiana	1992	Increase of Gamblers Anonymous groups	Campbell and Lester 1999	

Availability effects are best demonstrated in studies that compare changes in communities randomly assigned to adopt a policy change in availability with control communities, in other words, randomized controlled trials. These are rare in policy studies in general and so far absent in studies of gambling policies. A second best choice is the quasi-experimental design without random assignment of the policy intervention and control communities. A number of studies have applied a still simpler, uncontrolled design based on observed outcomes before and after the policy intervention in one site only, without controls. Such studies are commonly used to evaluate national policy changes, where a controlled study design may be difficult or even impossible to apply. Assessment of policy impact with uncontrolled study designs needs to pay particular attention

Table 7.2 Impact studies of reduced availability of gambling machines.

Country	Availability Change	Year	Outcomes	References	Observations
NORWAY	Temporary EGM prohibition; afterwards Norsk Tipping monopoly	2007	Problem gambling prevalence; differing results depending on measurement, but problem gambling help seeking decreased	Rossow and Hansen 2016; Lund 2009	Combined with EGM modifications, removal of note acceptors, personal identification card
SWITZERLAND	Gambling machines outside casinos prohibited	2005	No decrease in problem gambling, but clear reduction of problem gamblers with probable alcohol problem	Bondolfi et al. 2008	Same time permission to open 19 casinos
US	Temporary ban of EGMs in South Dakota	1994	Significant decrease of visits to problem gambling treatment facilities	Carr et al. 1996	Ban lasted only three months
US	Ban of EGMs in South Carolina	2000	Number and size of Gamblers Anonymous groups decreased	Bridwell and Quinn 2002, Williams et al. 2012b	Demand for help with problem gambling remained low in later years as well as during the ban.

to other factors that may have contributed to the observed changes. Finally, a number of studies have examined cross-regional co-variation in availability and gambling behavior and/or problem gambling. Such analyzes can rarely account for all other relevant factors contributing to cross-regional variation in gambling behavior and harms, and consequently findings from these studies may, at best, be considered as additional supportive information to other studies with stronger study designs.

Exposure to casinos

Most evaluation research on availability has been carried out on casinos, which often influence availability substantially for those living within easy reach. Williams et al. (2011b) observe in an extensive review that these changes in exposure to a casino pertain almost entirely to *increases* in availability. These studies mainly measure problems associated with gambling in a community before and after the opening of a casino. The Russian case presented in Box 7.1 is an exception. The prevalence of problem gambling (measured, for example, by the South Oaks Gambling Scale (SOGS)) seems to be the most common indicator of gambling problems. Other outcome measures include changes in crime, help seeking and suicide rates.

There is ample evidence, especially from the United States, Canada, and Australia, suggesting the negative impact of new casinos. The review by Williams and colleagues (2011b) shows that the majority of studies (22/33) found adverse outcomes of increased exposure to casinos. Similarly, the review by Tong and Chim (2013) of the relationship of casino proximity to problem gambling found a positive relationship in 7 of 11 studies. The studies discussed in the next paragraphs were selected because of their illustrative nature, wide scope or high quality.

Casinos and other gambling operations on American Indian reservations were legalized in many states in the United States subsequent to the Indian Gaming Regulatory Act of 1988. Las Vegas-style casinos with EGMs and table games were opened in many places, and this increase in availability was evaluated by Evans and Topoleski (2002). They found that four years after the casinos had opened, auto-theft, larceny, violent crime, and bankruptcy had all risen by about 10% in most cases.

Room and colleagues (1999) evaluated the effects of opening a casino in Niagara Falls, Ontario, a city on the Canadian side of the border with the United States. The goal was to attract gamblers from the United States, but the evaluation showed a local effect. Niagara Falls residents increased the number of positive responses to questions measuring past-year gambling problems (the short SOGS) by 51%. The residents' reports of gambling problems among their family and their friends also rose, by 46% (Room et al. 1999). A controlled study of the effects of another new casino opening in Canada (Jacques and Ladouceur 2006) distinguished between short term and longer term effects. The investigators found immediate (within one year of the opening) increases in gambling activity and gambling losses. These effects were not sustained in a follow-up study four years later. However, only one-quarter of the original sample was reached (203 cases in the test site). The result may have been affected by differential attrition of heavier gamblers from the sample. Meanwhile, the percentage of respondents reporting there was a problem gambler in their

Box 7.1 The 2006 gambling reform in Russia

After the dissolution of the Soviet Union in 1991, casinos and slot machine arcades mushroomed with few restrictions, and gambling started to have negative impacts on people's lives (Kassinove et al. 1998). In 1994, 496 gambling companies were registered. By 2006, the Russian authorities had given out 6,300 new licenses (Tsytsarev 2008).

Following negative media coverage of the Russian gambling industry in 2006 (Vasiliev and Bernhard 2012), a law was passed to ban gambling establishments and online gambling across the Russian territory, except for four 'gambling zones'. These zones were to be located at a distance from the major cities, in the Altai Territory (later replaced by Sochi), Primorye Territory, the Kaliningrad exclave, and on the border of the Krasnodar Territory and Rostov Region. In 2014, President Putin also proposed a bill to add a gambling zone in the Crimean Peninsula, following the Russian take-over of Crimea (Antonova 2014). Other gambling establishments and all online sites were ordered to be closed down by July 1, 2009. Only a limited number of bookmakers, betting shops, and charity lotteries are allowed outside the gambling zones. The Russian law was ambitious but inadequately prepared and badly implemented. The Kremlin chose the gambling zones but some of the local authorities were not happy with the decision (Haworth 2008). Authorities from the Altai and Kaliningrad territories asked to have the zones located elsewhere in order to protect their residents. Neither customers nor operators have been satisfied with the new zones. Russian gambling companies have invested abroad, often in locations easily accessible to Russian consumers such as Belarus (Vasiliev and Bernhard 2012). Inefficient enforcement may undermine the law's impact on problem gambling (Tsytsarev 2008). Illegal gambling remains widely available, and many former EGM halls now operate under the guise of internet cafés (Tarasov 2010). An interview study conducted in 2014 among 103 help-seeking problem gamblers in Moscow found that 90 participants played EGMs although they no longer are officially available in the city (Avtonomov 2014).

household had doubled by the fourth year in the test site, while declining in the control site.

In Sweden, the opening of casinos in two cities, Malmö and Sundsvall, was evaluated in a partially controlled study (Westfelt 2006). Malmö was chosen primarily to attract customers from neighboring Denmark, while the Sundsvall casino was expected to bring jobs to a depressed region. The volume of gambling increased in the first year in both cities after the casino openings, but a further rise was found at a three-year follow-up only in Malmö. Rates of current gambling problems (short SOGS and *DSM-IV*) increased after one year in both Malmö and Sundsvall, and further increased in both places in the three-year follow-up. These increases were matched in Malmö by answers to questions on problems with gambling among relatives and among friends, and in Sundsvall by answers on relatives but not on friends.

Several uncontrolled studies have compared rates of problem and pathological gambling before and after the opening of a casino. The introduction of casinos in four communities in Canada found that problem gambling rates increased in only one of the communities (Mangham et al. 2007). Another casino opening in the city of Windsor, Ontario, Canada, did not increase gambling expenditures, nor problem gambling rates after one year (Govoni et al. 1998). However, a four-year follow-up found that, while the rate of problem gambling among those who were gambling had not increased, the gambling participation rate in the population had increased, so that the rate of problem gamblers in the population as a whole had increased by more than one-third (Frisch 1999). Finally, a study from Switzerland (Bondolfi et al. 2008) found that the opening of 19 new casinos was not accompanied by a change in the prevalence of Problem and Pathological gambling. In this case, the casino openings had been tied to several compensatory preventive measures, including the prohibition of EGMs outside the casinos, and these measures may have neutralized the effects of the new casinos.

Other studies have found that casino openings were not accompanied by increased bankruptcies (Boardman and Perry 2007; Koo et al. 2007), crime rates (Johnson and Ratcliffe 2014; Koo et al. 2007), or suicide rates (McCleary et al. 2002). On the other hand, Grinols and Mustard (2006) estimated that between 5.5% and 30% of six different crimes (rape, robbery, aggravated assault, burglary, larceny, and auto theft) could be attributed to the presence of a casino. A number of cross-sectional studies have found associations between living near a casino and problem gambling (Welte et al. 2015; Williams et al. 2011b). Such correlations do not necessarily predict outcomes of policy changes, as other factors may explain them at least in part. For instance, casinos are often located in areas with a high proportion of problem gamblers or otherwise vulnerable persons, and people with gambling problems may choose to live close to a casino (Shaffer and Korn 2002). Casino employees have high problem rates, which may also influence these correlations (Williams et al. 2011b).

Some studies have considered the overall exposure to gambling in a jurisdiction. Welte et al. (2004a) found that people who lived within 16 kilometers of a casino were twice as likely to be problem gamblers as people who live further away. Gerstein et al. (1999) have also reported that in the United States, problem gambling rates within a 50-mile radius of a casino are twice as high as those at over 50 miles.

The general conclusion is that the association between casino gambling and harm rates is probably of modest to moderate magnitude. The establishment of a new casino increases gambling-related problems in the area; but casinos are also often set up in economically and socially deprived areas with vulnerable populations, and this may be a collateral factor (Goss and Morse 2009). Introducing new gambling opportunities in such communities should raise concerns about the consequences and alternative development strategies should be considered.

Some countries have abolished almost all casino operations. This has been the case in Turkey in 1998, Russia in 2006, and Ukraine in 2009. There have been no studies on the impacts of these changes, but it is clear that, as with most such prohibitions, one result is the continuation of some gambling illegally or offshore. For example, Northern Cyprus has been the great beneficiary of the Turkish ban on casinos, and has turned into a Las Vegas-type destination for Turkish gamblers. The Russian case is discussed in Box 7.1.

Availability of EGMs

Substantial research has been conducted on the availability of EGMs. As EGMs are the mainstay of most present-day casinos, these studies to some extent parallel research on casinos. A systematic review on the effects of proximity to and density of gambling machines found a positive but complex relationship between availability and gambling participation, expenditure, and especially, risk of problem gambling. Proximity appears to be more significant than density (Vasiliadis et al. 2013).

Increases in EGM availability have been studied particularly in Australia and New Zealand, where EGMs are highly available in residential areas. Beginning in 1991, EGMs were allowed in clubs and 'hotels' (bars) in Queensland, Australia. One study showed that EGM availability was accompanied by an increase in problem gambling (Australian Institute for Gambling Research 1995). Similar findings were reported from Tasmania, Australia (South Australian Centre for Economic Studies 2008). A meta-analysis of 34 population surveys of Australia and New Zealand between 1991 and 2007 (Storer et al. 2009) found that each additional EGM was associated with approximately 0.8 additional problem gamblers. However, Volberg and Abbott (2005) have suggested that there is a ceiling on this availability effect, with the linear relationship breaking down at around seven machines per 1,000 adults.

Apart from such case studies, other research has examined cross-sectional co-variation between EGM availability and outcome variables. Storer and colleagues (2009) found a moderate positive correlation between EGM density and problem gambling prevalence in the meta-analysis already described. A positive correlation between EGM density and problem gambling prevalence was found in data from Canadian provinces (Williams et al. 2012a). In Australia and New Zealand, regions with the highest density of EGMs have been associated with higher participation rates, spending rates, and problem gambling rates in EGM gambling than lower-density regions (Marshall 2005; Australian Productivity Commission 1999). Evidence from Australia and New Zealand has also shown that living a short distance to an EGM venue is associated with more spending and higher participation rates in gambling (Young et al. 2012; Pearce et al. 2008; Marshall and Wynne 2004). Wall and colleagues (2010) found that EGM availability in New Zealand was linked to crime rates; the closer the venue, the higher the crime rate. However, such correlations may also reflect other factors; for instance, EGMs are often concentrated in economically deprived neighborhoods (Marshall and Baker 2002; Robitaille and Herjean 2008; Rintoul et al. 2013), which may in part explain co-variations.

Many countries allow the government to regulate the number of EGMs located outside casinos. Policy experience in several countries suggests that accessibility rather than the sheer number of machines affects gambling behavior, but accessibility must be changed substantially to reduce gambling activity in contexts where it has already become common. Table 7.2 gives details of impact studies of reduced availability of gambling machines.

Reductions in EGM availability have been less frequent than increases, and their effects are less well documented. Temporary bans for a few months have been associated with drops in visits to problem gambling treatment facilities, in Gamblers Anonymous attendance, and in calls to a gamblers' helpline in several US states (Bridwell and Quinn 2002; Williams et al. 2012b). Studies from Australia and Canada (South Australian Centre for Economic Studies 2005; Delfabbro 2009; Corporate Research Associates 2006) have concluded that reductions in EGM numbers have an effect, but only if they are of considerable size. A reduction by 15% of EGMs in South Australia or by 5% in Victoria did not result in behavioral changes, whereas a reduction by 25% of the machines in Nova Scotia showed a decrease in both expenditure and time spent gambling. This would suggest that reductions have to be relatively significant to have an impact. Furthermore, in the Australian case, the machines that were removed were the least profitable and least popular (Vasiliadis et al. 2013).

Effects of the Norwegian EGM reforms 2001–2009

The substantial reduction and modification of EGM gambling in Norway, and its results, are exceptionally instructive. EGM gambling increased dramatically in Norway in the 1990s in response to technological developments and to simultaneous liberalization of gambling policy. Gross turnover on EGMs increased by a factor of 47 over a decade (Fekjær 2008, 77–78). A governmental gaming authority was established in 2001 and a state monopoly on EGMs was set up in 2003 (Rossow and Hansen 2016). Other restrictions on EGM gambling included bans on bank note acceptors (from July 1, 2006) and night opening (from January 1, 2007). A temporary ban on all EGMs was imposed from July 1, 2007. The monopoly introduced in 2009 a new type of less harmful EGMs with limited audio-visual stimuli, automatic game-abruption, no cash pay-out, and fixed upper limits for losses per day and per month. A mandatory personal gambling card helped to enforce minimum legal age and offered gamblers the options to restrict maximum losses and to impose self-exclusion. The new machines were placed in gas stations, kiosks, bars, and cafes, but their number was about one fifth of the pre-ban years (Rossow and Hansen 2016). The data derived from research on this natural experiment permits a high degree of confidence in conclusions about causal effects.

Figure 7.1 shows that gambling help line calls decreased significantly in the six months after the ban on bank note acceptors and decreased further after the ban on EGMs (Rossow and Hansen, 2016). Referrals to treatment decreased in a similar fashion after these restrictions (Engebø and Gyllstrøm 2008).

Prevalence of gambling problems in population surveys was lower after the EGM restrictions, with the exception of one problem gambling measure in youth (Rossow and Hansen 2016).

The restrictions also led to significant decreases in EGM turnover and total gambling. The ban on note acceptors led to a 17% reduction in gross turnover on EGMs and a net decrease in total gambling turnover by 10% for the entire year of 2006. The ban on night-time EGM gambling from January 1 and the temporary ban of EGMs from July 1 in 2007 led to a 55% reduction in EGM turnover and a net decrease in total gambling turnover by 28%. The turnover on all games decreased by 31% from 2007 to 2008. Since then, total gambling increased but did not return to the high of 2005, and EGM use remains below 25% of total gambling, instead of 60% in the period before the restrictions.

The Norwegian experience suggests that problems can be reduced by policies that restrict access to EGMs, though governments must accept that this is likely to decrease the monetary volume of the activity.

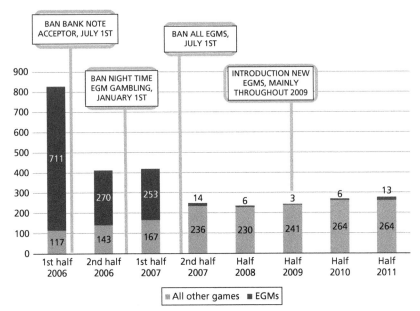

Fig 7.1 Number of help line calls per half year and main problem game
Reproduced from Engebø, J., and Gyllstrøm, F. (2008) Regulatory changes and finally a ban on existing slot machines in Norway: What's the impact on the market and problem gambling? 2008 International Gambling Conference, New Zealand. Available at https://hjelpelinjen.no/fakta-og-info/

There have been other dramatic changes in EGM availability in recent years. In Poland, EGMs were widely available in convenience locations until 2015, when a new law confined them in casinos and gambling halls. A similar development took place in Hungary in 2013, when convenience EGMs were forbidden and EGM gambling moved inside casinos (Szczyrba et al. 2016). There are not yet any evaluative studies on the impacts of these policy changes.

Physical access to other forms of gambling

Lotteries

Lotteries are generally considered to create fewer problems than continuous games. Nevertheless, negative effects of increased lottery availability have been reported. Average household gambling expenditures per week doubled after the introduction of the National Lottery in the United Kingdom in the mid-1990s, and the proportion of households with excessive expenditures (over 10% of household income) increased by a factor of four (Grun and McKeigue 2000). Gambling expenditures as a proportion of household income increased more in low income groups. This finding replicates observations from many countries that gambling constitutes a form of regressive taxation (Blalock et al. 2007;

Beckert and Lutter 2009; Freund and Morris 2005; Pirog-Good and Mikesell 1995; Tan and Yen 2010; Wiggins et al. 2010). Other studies of lottery availability and harm (e.g. crime rates and suicide rates) have produced mixed results (Williams et al. 2012b) and are not sufficient to establish a basis for policy conclusions.

Sports betting

Studies on sports betting and gambling problems are rare. Co-variation between sports betting venues (such as race tracks) and harm indicators (problem gambling rates, number of Gamblers Anonymous groups, and bankruptcies) has been studied, with mixed results (Pearce et al. 2008; Boardman and Perry 2007; Thalheimer and Ali 2004). There has also been mixed reporting on whether accessibility to sports betting venues is connected to demand (Mao 2013; Mao et al. 2015).

Internet gambling

Internet gambling is increasing globally, but it is still a minor fraction of the gambling market (see Chapter 3). Studies have shown that problem gambling rates are higher among online or mixed gamblers in comparison to land-based gamblers (Gainsbury et al. 2014b; Tovar et al. 2013; Wardle et al. 2011b) The introduction of an internet gambling license system in France was accompanied by increased overall gambling participation in the population (Costes et al. 2015). The prevalence of pathological gamblers (measured with the Canadian Problem Gambling Index (CPGI) scale) rose in the French population from 0.4% to 0.5% between 2010 (before the deregulation of the gambling market) and 2014. Problem gamblers increased from 1.3% to 2.2% (Costes et al. 2015). Conversely, in Germany internet gambling was reduced after its prohibition in 2008 (Ludwig et al. 2012).

In a 2013 national sample of the French population (n = 4,042), problem gambling prevalence was higher than average in online environments: 6.6% of online gamblers displayed a high risk of gambling problems, 10.4% a moderate risk, and 23.8% a low risk (Tovar et al. 2013).

A Spanish study (Chóliz 2016) with pathological gamblers in recovery (n = 1,277) found that online gambling was second only to EGMs as the main cause for pathological gambling. This was remarkable because at the time of the data collection, online gambling had only been legally available for a few months.

Higher problem gambling rates among online gamblers have been attributed to availability (Gainsbury et al. 2014b). However, Philander and Mackay (2014) found that the availability of online gambling does not increase problem gambling per se, but those who participate have other characteristics that may make them more vulnerable than land-based gamblers. A common finding has been that online players include more young males and have higher educational levels compared to gamblers in land-based venues (e.g. Griffiths et al. 2009a; Tovar et al. 2013; Australian Productivity Commission 2010). Furthermore, smart phones and other mobile devices are the most accessible gambling platform. Drakeford and Hudson Smith (2015) talk about instant accessibility. Opening hours and proximity are no longer the key issue with mobile gambling, but rather the constant attachment to a device that receives notifications and advertising to keep playing. The regulation of online gambling varies considerably across jurisdictions (Williams et al. 2012c). The options are similar across the world: prohibition, state monopoly, licensing, and open market. These are usually applied in combination. For example, offering online wagering is lawful in Australia for licensed operators. However, offering non-wagering games (e.g., slots, casino games) is not permitted by the 'Interactive Gambling Act.' International sites are widely accessed but the policy may have reduced the volume of participation (Australian Productivity Commission 2010). Blocking access to a website is the most common and direct form of regulation, but it can be circumvented easily, and maintenance of a list of blocked sites requires significant resources. Only a few suggestive findings on policy effectiveness are available.

Policy effectiveness depends on the effort and willingness of public authorities to control the trade. In the absence of any international agreement (see Chapter 10), their only recourse is to try to control the internet or its providers, or to control financial institutions paying or transferring money—either by direct measures, or by threatening other interests of non-cooperative providers. One way to control the internet, used for instance in China, is to block access to blacklisted websites. This can be achieved either through Domain Name System (DNS) filtering or Internet Protocol (IP) blocking. DNS filtering is the more popular approach (European Commission 2012), and is used for example in France and Quebec. The problem with this technique is that keeping the database up to date requires resources, and blocks are easy to circumvent. Despite its large investment in controlling domestic internet access, China has struggled to control internet gambling, as indicated in March 2017 by the Public Security Minister, who said that police "must root out criminal gangs operating online gambling and show no mercy to 'underground banks' which aid with the flow of cash to cross-border betting" (Yan 2017).

The US government has had some success with controlling financial institutions which pay or transfer money after the Unlawful Internet Gambling Enforcement Act in 2006 and the earlier Wire Act adopted in 1968 (Department of Social Services 2015). Payment blocking is used also in France, Norway, and Germany. American payment service providers are responsible under criminal law for preventing unauthorized gambling payments.

German transactions for online gambling are not allowed, but payment service providers are not liable under criminal law (Fiedler 2016b). Norway has the most experience with this kind of measure in Europe. Internet gambling is limited by law but payment blocking has not fulfilled the initial expectations (Rossow and Hansen 2016). Also payment blocks can be circumvented by using online payment services. The European Commission (2012) has noted that in countries where payment blocks have been introduced, consumers have moved on to unlicensed gambling websites where they can use their credit cards. Some credit card companies like American Express avoid this by refusing to accept gambling transactions at all.

Country-specific domain names are mandatory in France and Spain (European Commission 2012). The regulation of internet gambling still remains a national issue, as financial interests of the individual EU member states are at stake (Laffey et al. 2016). A further option is to use criminal sanctions against unlicensed providers, but this approach is difficult and costly to enforce, particularly for providers with no presence or assets in the country.

Restrictions on who can gamble

Availability of gambling can be restricted by setting limits on who can gamble. These limits mainly entail minimum age. Most jurisdictions have placed age limits on gambling, usually varying between 15 and 21 years depending on the location and type of game (Williams et al. 2012b). In many European countries, the minimum age for all gambling has been raised from 15 or 16 to 18 following the increasing attention the European Commission has paid to consumer protection in gambling (European Commission 2012). Alcohol studies have shown that age limits are an effective tool (e.g., Babor et al. 2010), but few studies have been conducted regarding gambling. Available results are nevertheless encouraging. In Finland, the legal age limit for EGM gambling was raised from 15 to 18 in 2011. An evaluative study of the policy change (Raisamo et al. 2015b) showed that prevalence of EGM use among 12–16-year olds declined from 44% in 2011 to 13% in 2013. Similar results were reported in Norway after the minimum age of participation was raised from 16 to 18 (Götestam and Johansson 2009). Youth gambling prevalence studies also show that in jurisdictions with age restrictions for gambling, adolescents gamble less (Calado et al. 2016).

Other restrictions on who can gamble include self-exclusions and other exclusion policies that are discussed in Chapter 9. Several governments stipulate that local residents cannot gamble at the casino in their community (Williams et al. 2012b). Such rules have been applied in some Asian countries (Williams et al. 2012b). One example is South Korea, where citizens are only allowed to gamble at one of the nation's 16 casinos. Participation in casino gambling, as well as the prevalence of problem gambling, is considerably lower than in other Asian jurisdictions (Williams et al. 2013). In the Monte Carlo casino in Monaco, local citizens have been banned from gambling or working at the casino since its mid-19th century inception. Such regulations are becoming less common because they require identity checks at entry. Nevertheless, many governments allow casinos only on sites close to borders or in tourist destinations.

Temporal restrictions

Many jurisdictions have restrictions on the opening hours of gambling venues. The most interesting policy experiences on restricting opening hours come from Australia, where restrictions on EGM venue opening hours have been introduced in the 2000s. Evaluative studies have been conducted in Victoria, the Australian Capital Territory, and New South Wales after venues were no longer permitted to remain open for 24 hours (South Australian Centre for Economic Studies 2005; McMillen and Pitt 2005; New South Wales 2003). These studies found minor or no impact following a mandatory three-hour shutdown, implemented during early morning hours. In Nova Scotia, Canada, a longer shutdown after midnight showed a more significant impact, reducing net gambling revenue by 5–9% and spending by problem gamblers by 18% (Nova Scotia Gaming Corporations 2005). This evidence suggests that temporal restrictions should be substantial in order to have an impact.

Price and cost

It has long been recognized that raising the costs for consumers to involve themselves in problematic health behaviors is one of the most efficient instruments to promote public health. By contrast, gamblers seldom have a clear view of what the cost of participation is. In fact, as shown elsewhere in this book, gambling designers intentionally obfuscate the actual cost of participation with illusionary winning chances, maintaining arousal with near wins, auditory and visual stimuli, and other techniques.

Losing money in the long run is inevitable for nearly anyone gambling in a commercial market. The 'house take' is the part left with the game provider after reduction of the returns to the players. It is generally shared among three parties: the provider of the game, the state (in the form of a tax or license fee), and sometimes also a 'good cause' in whose name or for whose benefit the game is being run. The state's portion in the form of taxes and fees varies considerably between forms of gambling. In Australia in 1995–1996, for instance, the state's take on the turnover (that is, on a base of the net expenditure) was 82% for lotteries, 37% for racing bets, 27% for EGMs, and 20% for casinos (Smith 2000).

Buying a lottery ticket thus only makes rational sense if a high price is accepted for the value of dreaming. Governments' interest in setting prices for gambling by taxes and other means is usually driven by the revenue motive alone, without attention to effects on the problematic consequences of the activity. Furthermore, gambling proceeds designated for good purposes that are included in the 'price' of participation are often outside governments' control, as they are delivered by operators directly as contributions towards such uses.

Substantial evidence indicates that EGM gamblers are not sensitive to price, given the difficulty in conceptualizing price on an EGM, and in ascertaining it. The Australian Productivity Commission (1999) noted that demand was most likely price inelastic (i.e., consumers would not change behavior when prices rose) because of lack of price information and lack of substitutability. Evidence for the latter is that although lower 'priced' table games are readily available in casinos, users continue to use EGMs, which may cost as much as ten times the 'price' of a table game (Australian Productivity Commission 1999).

During a period of intense competition in EGM operations in Victoria (1992–2012), one operator set the 'price' of EGM use at a lower level than their competitor. The only effect was to suppress revenue for the 'cheaper' operator. After a period of five years the 'price' of EGM games offered by the operators converged (Woolley et al. 2013). There is little evidence that EGM users can detect price differentials, although in extreme experimental studies (where the price of the game is varied substantially) there is some evidence that users can detect this (Dixon et al. 2013). In any event, price as a concept is difficult to apply in the gambling market, especially in the case of EGMs.

Still, some studies show that price influences the gambling consumer's behavior, and price elasticities of demand have been calculated. Defined as the ratio of the percentage change in gambling demand to the percentage change in price, the mean price elasticity reported in the literature is about -1, i.e., a 10% rise in price would produce a 10% fall in purchasing of the gambling product—but with a substantial range in the elasticities (standard deviation 0.73). Analyzing 46 price elasticity studies in a meta-analysis, Gallet (2015) found that the demand for casino gaming tends to be less responsive to price than the demands for horse racing and for lotteries. Lottery demand tended to be about -1. Price elasticities for Europe and Asia tended to fall in the elastic range, while for the United States they generally fell in the inelastic range, suggesting that a multinational firm could earn greater profits for a given level of effort in the United States than in Europe or Asia.

Although gamblers playing on an EGM or buying a lottery ticket are often uninformed about the odds on their game, the elasticity studies show that their behavior is influenced by the cost of their participation. Many countries mandate a minimum return percentage to maintain some sort of standard integrity of games (Harrigan and MacLaren 2014). Some gambling providers, such as the French national lottery, even justify their low return percentages as a harm reduction strategy. High return percentages cause less financial loss but they may also produce more rewards that reinforce gambling behavior. Research remains inconclusive regarding whether high return levels encourage problem gambling (Parke and Parke 2013). It is possible that a certain return range is connected to problem gambling, allowing enough rewards for the player but also significant profits for the operator. Such a return percentage is probably around the range of 75% to 92% that is found in most EGMs (Williams et al. 2012b).

Governments have the opportunity to reduce gambling overall or to suppress a particular form of gambling. They can also raise taxes on all forms of gambling. This works to a limited extent directly, making spending less attractive to players. A more powerful mechanism is to make gambling offers less profitable to providers, thus reducing their interest in expanding the market. A key issue is transparency and the provision of reliable information on the actual rate of losses to the gamblers. Regulating the price of the activity by implementing taxes or levies is likely to fail as a measure to reduce gambling unless the levies are so high that the whole industry in one particular area or location is affected.

Conclusions

Research generally finds that large-scale changes in availability, either up or down, have substantial effects on levels of gambling, of problem gambling, and of harms from gambling. With smaller-scale changes, the results are more variable, reflecting the interplay with other factors. The literature mostly refers to changes in the direction of increased access to gambling. The few restrictive regulations referred to in the literature have often coincided with other regulatory changes (as in Norway, Switzerland, and Germany), which makes it hard to isolate availability effects from other factors. Evidence on the effects of price on consumer behavior is inconclusive, but it can be firmly asserted that higher taxes and fees, if applied consistently, reduce the attractiveness of the field to operators.

There is a need for more studies on gambling availability changes, preferably with control sites for comparison. These studies should look beyond measuring only prevalence of problem gambling scores as an outcome. Such scores often yield quite low rates in general population samples, and are thus very sensitive to sample size and measurement errors. Evaluations of availability impacts should ideally build on a host of other outcome measures, including total gross gaming revenue changes, distribution of expenditures, measures of harm in different population groups, and harm experienced by gamblers' families, workplaces, and communities.

Usually availability changes are small and their effects are therefore difficult to detect even in carefully planned study designs. When changes in many outcome measures are in the same direction, inferences of intervention impact can be drawn more safely. In this respect, the Norwegian policy experiences of a temporary ban in EGMs followed by the re-introduction of new machines provides a compelling example of a likely causal relationship between availability restrictions and reduced harms.

Chapter 8

Industry strategies and their regulation: marketing, game features, and venue characteristics

As in other commercial activities, gambling providers aim to gain a profit to owners, often accompanied by an extra share of returns for public use. The profits can be increased by attracting more gamblers, by keeping them in the gambling occasion for more time, and by inducing them to spend more. An important aim is keeping intensive players "in the zone". Gamblers use this term to describe an altered state of consciousness where the worries and expectations of the world fade away. Electronic gambling machines (EGMs) especially allow some players to escape into a state of other-worldliness where mundane pre-occupations cease to be important (Woolley and Livingstone 2010). Removal from the diurnal world is typically reinforced by the absence of windows and clocks in casinos and gaming rooms.

Much of the knowledge on game inducement is in the hands of the industry. Researchers and policymakers have fewer resources to conduct studies on the same factors, and are often left with evaluating and analyzing undesirable effects of already implemented strategies. Available evidence concerns high-intensity gambling on EGMs, in casinos, and in online gambling environments. This chapter accordingly concentrates on these contexts, in which "reverse-engineering" of industry strategies for public interest purposes has been most developed (e.g., Schüll 2012). It focuses on three industry strategies that can be regulated and used as policy levers: marketing, game features, and venue characteristics. Experiences of regulating these features will be summarized in the last section.

Marketing

Marketing operates by offering inspiration, cues, and confirmation of initial intentions to participate in gambling activities. It aims to recruit new gamblers, to intensify regular gamblers' participation, and it may cause re-lapses. The power of marketing is greatest in societies where new consumers can be recruited, and in immature rather than mature markets (Binde 2007b; 2014). Almost all countries have legislation requiring "truth in advertising", and many countries have introduced additional control techniques specific to this area (Williams et al. 2012b). As the gambling experience depends on im-agination, hope, and other intangible factors, this truthfulness requirement is difficult to enforce, and marketing practices importunately test and push the limits of such legislation.

Prevalence of marketing

In some countries gambling marketing contributes significantly to advertise-ment revenue of the media. In the United Kingdom it accounts for about 4% of all televised advertisement (Ofcom 2013), and up to 11% on certain internet sites (Sandberg et al. 2011). Restrictions vary from a total ban to more or less controls. Typically, advertisement is allowed only for domestically licensed operators (Williams et al. 2012b). Rules vary between games and providers. The promotion of national lotteries, in particular, enjoys a public legitimacy, while advertisement of commercial casinos may be illegal in the same context (Griffiths 2005). Advertisement of national monopolies has even been justified in terms of harm-reduction, as the promotion of relatively harmless gambling opportunities may steer consumption away from more dangerous products (Binde 2014).

Online technology has provided new marketing tools. These include site-advertising and pop-up windows as well as e-mail and phone messages. Profiling enables targeted advertisement to certain population groups.

Targeting vulnerable groups

There is convincing evidence that problem gamblers are particularly sensitive to promotion: they are likely to be more positively influenced, but also more likely to act on cues (Williams et al. 2012b; Hing et al. 2013). Interview studies have found that advertisement undermines intentions to reduce or to stop playing (Planzer and Wardle 2011; Binde 2009).

Advertising targeted at adolescents is prohibited in many countries. Studies have found that adolescents are easily influenced by advertisements even when they are able to judge critically its content (Monaghan et al. 2008). Interview studies report that exposure generates positive images of gam-bling (Derevensky et al. 2009) and increases intentions to gamble (Felsher et al 2003).

Marketing content

Marketing research distinguishes between objectively and subjectively misleading advertising. Intentionally and objectively deceitful marketing is often defined as illegal by general advertising codes. Subjectively misleading marketing displays emotionally charged misrepresentations of winning with spurious images of skill. Lottery advertisement in particular appeals to winning as a life-changing chance (Monaghan et al. 2008) and downplays or conceals the actual odds (McMullan and Miller 2009). In some countries, lotteries are presented as beneficial to society due to their part in collecting public funds (Korn et al. 2005).

Casino and online gambling advertisements typically connect gambling to excitement, instant gratification, and glamour, while at the same time suggesting that casino gambling is a normal pastime (Monaghan 2008; McMullan and Miller 2008 2010) or even a family-friendly leisure activity (Youn et al. 2000).

Sports sponsorship visually embeds gambling advertisement in arenas and in media diffusion of the sporting event, often associating gambling products with sport celebrities and images of good health (Thomas et al. 2012).

Game features

Game features are developed to encourage and to prolong the gambling experience. A significant number of studies have measured the impact of bet and win sizes, theoretical loss, and other particular features on persistence, time spent in gambling, and levels of arousal (Griffiths 1993). EGMs have received the most attention, as they include more high intensity characteristics than any other form of gambling. Box 8.1 describes the strategies used by EGM designers to maximize the profits generated for game operations.

Payments, pay-outs, and credit displays

Payments, pay-outs, and credit displays can distance the player from real money. Bill acceptors, gambling chips, and electronic payments encourage players to spend more than was originally intended. In some jurisdictions, gamblers can insert debit or credit cards directly into EGMs. Research shows that the less abstraction there is regarding money wagered, the less risky gambling becomes. Gamblers tend to play more when playing with chips than with real money (Lapuz and Griffiths 2010). Converting money to credits on EGM display screens contributes to misjudgements about the amounts of money spent (Griffiths 1993). EGM players consider cash displays more helpful than credit displays in controlling their gambling (Schellinck and Schrans 2002; Wynne and Stinchfield 2004; Ladouceur and Sévigny 2009).

Box 8.1 Inside an Australian EGM: complexity in the service of ignorance

The price of using EGMs is the wager minus the amount that the game will return on average to the player. This is called the *return to player ratio* (RTP), or the total wager minus the "house edge". This is determined by the "game maths" but it is very difficult for the user to perceive.

> Typically, the machine features that are most lucrative to the operator entail many of the most problematic reinforcement characteristics such as high event frequency, interactive options, near wins, note acceptors or playing with credit cards, and encouraging sensory effects (Williams et al. 2012b).

Bet sizes

Some evidence suggests that large bet sizes increase arousal in players (Parke et al. 2014). Problem gamblers stake larger bets than recreational gamblers (Sharpe et al. 2005). Nonetheless, research has shown that limitations on bet sizes have to be significant to have an impact. A policy introduced in Australia to limit EGM bets to a maximum of ten dollars did not have any effect on gambling behavior (McMillen and Pitt 2005). However, an observational study showed that when machines were modified to allow maximum bets of one dollar instead of ten, time and money spent on gambling decreased (Sharpe et al. 2005).

On the other hand, EGM development has shifted to low bets with high event frequencies to increase *time on device* (Schüll 2012). A Norwegian study (Leino et al. 2015) used tracking data of EGM player activity (n = 31,109). Results showed that a lower maximum bet size actually *increased* gambling participation. The different empirical results may be due to insufficient reductions in bet size, but can also indicate that reducing bet sizes may have unintended consequences. Existing evidence seems to suggest that reducing bet sizes should be coupled with other measures to limit the total amount of spending.

Wins, losses, and return percentages

The size and frequency of wins and losses affect gambling behavior, but research has not been able to determine price thresholds for risky behavior (Parke and Parke 2013). Rockloff and colleagues (2015) tested in a laboratory study (n = 130) a pop-up message telling players that the jackpot has expired. Results showed that after viewing the jackpot expiry message, betting

Box 8.1 Inside an Australian EGM: complexity in the service of ignorance

(continued)

speed significantly slowed down and players were more likely to quit playing than in the control groups. The attractiveness of certain types of wins seems to depend on the game. Lottery players are particularly attracted by large rollover jackpots (Barclay 2007; Beenstock and Haitovsky 2001). Customers are most attracted to high jackpot EGMs (Williams et al. 2012b), but players appear to prefer pre-determined over progressive jackpots (Li et al. 2015).

Frequent small wins (Leino et al. 2015; Delfabbro and Winefield 1999) as well as losing streaks (Harris and Parke 2015) have been found to encourage EGM play. Data on 31,000 Norwegian EGM gamblers showed that small wins maintained gambling, whereas larger wins tended to disrupt it (Leino et al. 2015). There is evidence that problem gamblers are more motivated to continue gambling after a large win than recreational gamblers (Young et al. 2008).

At the heart of the EGM are random number generators. When the device is activated, numbers are generated at a speed measured in nano-seconds. The computer reads the numbers and uses these to display the outcome on the screen. The game mathematics are used to optimize the attractiveness of the game by using two factors:

- reel strips—the number and order of symbols on each virtual reel; and
- pay tables—the prizes awarded for each combination of symbols appearing on a line of the game on which a bet has been laid.

EGMs have a very large number of potential outcomes, frequently as many as 50,000,000 or more. The *Dolphin Treasure* game, a relatively old Australian-style EGM game, has 35,640,000 possible outcomes (Harrigan et al. 2014). To check the returns of all outcomes would require a minimum of 3.4 years of continuous use at game intervals of 5 seconds per spin.

The "house edge" for Australian-style EGMs is generally between 8% and 15% of the total amount of dollars spent on the machine. It is difficult to observe this ratio in the short term as it varies significantly from session to session.

Many users believe that if the game is operated in a fair manner, they should leave gambling venues with an amount consistent with the return to player ratio advertised—that is, with 85% to 92% of their stake. In fact, the total "price" calculation is the deduction of the price factor for each spin. If a user inserts AUD 10 and wagers one dollar each spin at a speed of five seconds, the user's funds would be exhausted in a little more than five minutes, even if the game performs exactly as predicted by the average (this is extremely unlikely). At five dollar bets this process would occupy a little over one minute.

> **Box 8.1 Inside an Australian EGM: complexity in the service of ignorance**
> *(continued)*
>
> The Australian Productivity Commission (1999 p.U11) undertook a calculation of mean and median time on device with the (then) well known game *Black Rhino*. Their calculation based on a 30 dollar stake, 1.50 dollar wagers and 5 second spins, was that average time on the game was 13 minutes and 4 seconds, with median time of less than 4 minutes. The difference between mean and median time results from a few exceptionally long play runs that push up the average.
>
> The playing style of users will influence time on the device. If a user bets only one credit on one line, time on the game may be longer compared to the examples in the above paragraph. However, most experienced EGM users employ a 'mini-max' or similar strategy (Harrigan et al. 2014; Livingstone et al. 2008), whereby they will select multiple lines (often as many as possible) and bet the minimum on each line. This means that fewer "winning" lines will be missed. It also makes "losses disguised as wins" possible.
>
> Game designers need to consider which strategy serves the operator best. It is possible to program the devices to maximize the turnover of customers by exhausting their funds quickly; on the other hand, they might lose customers who seek to "stay in the zone". Computerized casinos and online games make it possible to adjust the machines according to demand, so that in slack periods players can stay on a device longer than in busy hours. In the end, however, only the house wins.

Equipping EGMs with note acceptors increases the convenience of play for gamblers, as well as revenue for providers (Williams et al. 2012b). The Australian Productivity Commission (1999) showed that 65% of problem gamblers use note acceptors, as opposed to only 23% of recreational gamblers.

Policy experiences with removing note acceptors have shown promising results. In Norway, a 2006 ban on note acceptors resulted in a 24% decrease in the number of people seeking help for gambling problems and a 17% decrease in gambling turnover (Rossow and Hansen 2016; Götestam and Johansson 2009). A Norwegian survey study (Hansen and Rossow 2010) conducted among 13–19-year-old Norwegians (n = 20,000) before and after the ban shows that the measure reduced both problem gambling and overall gambling participation among adolescents by 20%.

Sensory effects

Sounds, lights, and space are reinforcement techniques that make the player continue gambling. Sound and image engineering produces musical scores, complex sound effects, and verbal interaction (Parke and Griffiths 2006). Studies of regulation of these features have been few, but the prevalence of sensory effects in games does indicate industry knowledge on their importance in retaining players in gambling situations.

Evidence on sound effects is relatively conclusive. They heighten emotional states by creating an exciting gambling environment (Griffiths and Parke 2005; Bramley and Gainsbury 2014). According to laboratory evidence (Dixon et al. 2014), reinforcement sounds arouse players and make them overestimate their winnings. Even sounds coming from other machines have the potential to increase gambling intensity (Wolfson and Case 2000). An experimental study has reported that removing sounds decreased excitement and tension in players (Loba et al. 2001). Figure 8.1 shows the sensory characteristics of a New Zealand "pokie".

Illumination and visual complexity have also been studied. The color of light has been reported to have no impact on the numbers of bets or amounts of bets (Spenwyn et al. 2010), but the intensity of the lighting seems to have some effect. An experiment which lowered the illumination of EGMs by 35% increased the number of plays or the time playing (Delfabbro et al. 2005).

Interactive features

Gamblers often erroneously believe that they can recover losses from EGMs if they continue to play. They also tend to underestimate their spending due to random pay-outs and rapid repetition. According to the Australian Productivity Commission (2010), machine gamblers estimated their losses at around 3% of the real total. This may be because players conceal their losses from themselves or in reporting, but also because machines encourage faulty illusions of skill.

Illusion of skill is important for play encouragement (Parke and Griffiths 2006). A Norwegian population survey (n = 4,963) found that increased gambling frequency was associated with irrational beliefs, and the link was strongest for EGMs, card games, and online gambling (Lund 2011). These games encourage faulty cognitions to a more significant extent than non-continuous games such as weekly lotteries.

EGMs can easily be modified to incorporate features that increase false perceptions. These include bonuses, complex game boards, prize ladders, and the possibility to select the number of lines bet (Harrigan et al. 2014; Parke and Griffiths 2006). A large number of play lines increases operant reinforcement as

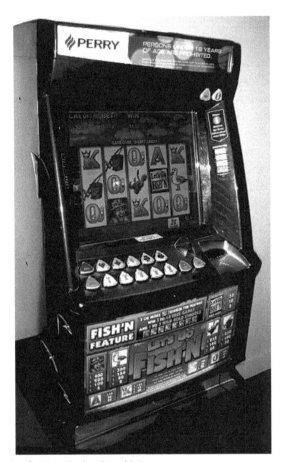

Fig 8.1 Example of a New Zealand "pokie"
Photograph by Alan Liefting.

well as the number of games played and time spent gambling (Harrigan et al. 2011; Delfabbro et al. 2005). Some Australian states have imposed constraints on play lines, but the numbers have remained high, with a maximum of 50 lines permitted in Queensland and 30 lines in Tasmania (Williams et al. 2012b).

Stop buttons give the illusion of being able to freeze lines in EGM play. A laboratory study among non-problem EGM gamblers in Canada (n = 48) (Ladouceur and Sévigny 2005) found that 87% of players believed that the use of the stop button would bring about different symbols on the screen, and 57% believed that they could influence the outcome.

Interactive characteristics are common in non-continuous and low-intensity forms of gambling. Sports betting attracts players with fixed or pool bets

(Hayer and Meyer 2005). Magical beliefs are commonly held about particular lottery numbers (Griffiths and Wood 2001; Davis et al. 2000; Ladouceur and Mayrand 1987).

Online gambling environments have characteristics that reinforce the interactive nature of games. This is particularly the case with practice sites and practice modes that attract gamblers by providing inflated return rates (Sévigny et al. 2005; Blaszczynski et al. 2001). Experimental evidence shows that players exposed to inflated return rates in the practice mode place higher bets than control groups in the real play mode (Frahn et al. 2015).

Speed

Speed of play is an integral part of EGM design, but also relevant in other games such as online gambling and instant lotteries. Speed depends on event frequency. Event frequency is the time elapsed between bet and final outcome. Australian EGMs run at the speed of above 600 events per hour; roulettes and blackjacks range from 50 to 100; and races below 20 events (Australian Productivity Commission 2010). Some jurisdictions mandate a minimum time gap in EGM events, ranging from 2.1 seconds in Victoria to 5 seconds in Spain (Williams et al. 2012b). Speed can be accelerated by replacing handles with buttons and by introducing touch screens, video technology, bill and banking card acceptors (Schüll 2012; Livingstone and Adams 2011). In some countries, autoplay features are added to machines (Parke and Griffiths 2006). Victoria, South Australia and Western Australia have banned the feature as it is presumed to cause harm (Williams et al. 2012b).

Speed can increase participation in other games besides EGMs. Griffiths and Wood (2001) have called scratch tickets "paper EGMs" as they have short pay-out intervals, high event frequencies, and the possibility to re-gamble winnings almost immediately. Scratch tickets can often be bought directly from dispensers, increasing the resemblance to EGMs. The Tactilo terminals in Switzerland move a step further, with tickets scratched electronically on an EGM-like machine (Villeneuve and Pasquier 2011).

Near misses and losses disguised as wins

A near miss refers to a situation which the player perceives as coming close to winning. These situations are very common in scratch cards and EGMs. According to some calculations, near misses lead the bettor to expect a return percentage between 192 and 1000% (Schüll 2012). Quasi-wins, also known as losses disguised as wins (LDWs), are a similar phenomenon, and typical in Australian-style pokies (EGMs). Machines operating LDWs pay something frequently, but usually less than the initial bet (Schüll 2012). The perception of a win is underscored, as the machine still celebrates the 'win' with all the lights and sounds that this entails (Harrigan and MacLaren 2014; Schüll 2012).

Near misses encourage faulty cognitions, motivate further play, and have a similar conditioning effect as a win (Parke and Griffiths 2004). They also create the same physiological and neural reactions in players (e.g., Clark et al. 2012; Qi et al. 2011). Most empirical evidence comes from laboratories with EGM types of gambling. Results have shown that players exposed to near misses play more and with higher bets than after real wins (Kassinove and Schare 2001; Côté et al. 2003).

Venue characteristics

Venue design is a method that operators employ to make gamblers play more but also to attract visitors who play with low intensity. Research has also identified some design elements that may be more problematic than others from the point of view of high risk-taking. Casinos use a variety of reinforcing stimuli from lights and sounds to croupiers' calls and jackpot signs. Immersive interiors, lack of daylight and clocks, as well as the service of alcohol are means to disorient gamblers' sense of space and time.

Casino design

European casinos typically function under a variety of restrictions concerning opening hours, house credit, advertisement and provision of alcoholic beverages. In contrast, American-type casinos have few restrictions on operating hours or other amenities (Thompson 2010; Chambers 2011). There have been no comparative studies between these models, but the lower rates of problem gambling in Europe may indicate that the European model has more consumer protection potential.

Some specific features in casino and gambling venue design may encourage gambling. A survey study (Hing and Haw 2010) found that recreational players considered extended opening hours to be the only problematic venue characteristic. Problem gamblers mentioned as risk factors: easy access to cash dispensers, a large repertoire of different machines, a private layout, and an atmosphere of glitz and glamour. A study from Québec showed that 74% of the participating players (n = 180) thought that playing EGMs in isolated cubicles was more problematic than in open space (Ladouceur et al. 2005).

Studies have shown that customers prefer casinos with high ceilings and clear lines (the so-called Krane playground model, Figure 8.2) to low ceilings and a compartmentalized décor (the Friedman model) (Finlay et al. 2007; 2010). According to one study, the Krane model encourages high-risk gambling to

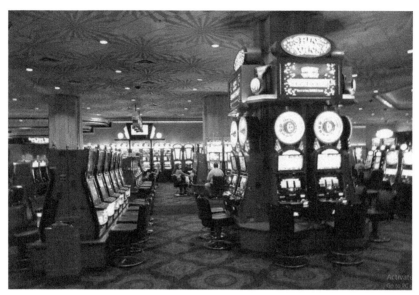

Fig 8.2 Electronic Gambling Machines organized according to Krane's model layout at the MGM Grand in Las Vegas
Photograph by Laslovarga, distributed under a CC BY-SA 3.0 license.

a larger degree than the Friedman model (Finlay et al. 2010). This may be because playing in larger crowds intensifies gambling behavior (e.g., Rockloff et al. 2011).

A number of studies have looked at the design of online gambling environments. Online poker sites use a diverse set of rhetorical, psychological, and immersive techniques to sell poker as an attractive consumer product (McMullan and Kervin 2012). Some websites borrow features from video games to immerse the player into the game and to tempt underage players (Paloheimo 2010; Friend and Ladd 2009). The evidence on online gambling designs still remains limited, but it appears that online operators use immersive 'spatial' design choices similar to land-based casinos.

Soundscape, lights, and clocks

Casino designers attempt to find the right balance between not assaulting players and not going completely unnoticed (Schüll 2012). Background music can increase gambling intentions (Harvey et al. 2007) but the tempo of music does not have an impact (Bramley 2015). In general, ambient casino sounds increase gambling intensity (Noseworthy & Finlay 2009; Brevers et al. 2015). Venues often change background music to match customer demographics (Griffiths and Parke 2005). Casino interiors are typically dark and lack natural light. Nearly one half of the respondents of an Australian survey thought that the introduction of natural light or a clock would be an effective measure to reduce harm (Rodda and Cowie 2005). Some laboratory experiments have shown that static light yields lower levels of intent to gamble than flashing lights (Finlay et al. 2010) and that gamblers play faster under red light than normal light (Brevers et al. 2015). However, a Canadian study (Wynne and Stinchfield 2004) found that adding on-screen clocks on EGMs has no impact on gambling behavior. Clocks may be yet another feature that is more likely to help recreational players avoid problems than those who already gamble excessively.

Inducements, alcohol, and smoking

Casinos provide loyalty programmes that reward customers with prizes and bonuses, or with access to various perks, such as free meals, hotel rooms, and chips for gambling (Eadington 1999). Loyalty programmes successfully encourage people to gamble more (Williams et al. 2012b). Inducements are also given for online gambling. Sites offer registration bonuses that are often accompanied by various conditions to play and deposit money (Sévigny et al. 2005). Inducements encourage player engagement, but their actual effect on gambler behavior or problem gambling is still unknown.

The evidence regarding the impact of the opportunity to smoke or consume alcohol while gambling is solid. Both alcohol and tobacco use has been connected to increased gambling, and alcohol use disorder and smoking are co-morbid with problem gambling (Baron and Dickerson 1999; Petry and Oncken 2002). Smoking bans at gambling locations have been introduced in many countries to protect employees from passive smoking, and not primarily as a gambling harm minimization strategy. Inadvertently, the policy has also been effective in reducing excessive gambling. Smoking bans have led to significant decreases in gambling revenues (see Williams et al. 2012b; Lal and Siahpush 2008) but revenue levels may recover after the initial dip. The recovery may be a result of smoking bans encouraging non-smokers to enter casinos, or because operators circumvent the policy by installing smoking rooms in the vicinity of games or inventing arrangements that allow them to define gambling rooms as "outside".

Casinos in the United States offer free alcoholic drinks, whereas Canada, New Zealand, and most European countries prohibit free or discounted alcoholic beverages in gambling locations (Williams et al. 2012b). In Chile, customers are not allowed to drink at all in gambling rooms (Thompson 2010). Limiting the availability of alcohol may be an effective harm reduction strategy because alcohol consumption intensifies play (Ellery et al. 2005; Kyngdon and Dickerson 1999), and the effect of alcohol has been found to be strong among problem gamblers (Ellery and Stewart 2014; Markham et al. 2012).

Access to funds

Casinos may allow players to access additional funds through on-site ATMs (Automatic Teller Machines accessing banks and credit cards), EFTPOS terminals (Electronic Fund Transfer Point of Sale, accessing debit cards) or house credit, but these are not allowed in some jurisdictions. Australian research has shown that venue-based ATMs are among the top causes for overspending among EGM players, and that large ATM withdrawals are more common among problem gamblers than non-problem gamblers (McMillen et al. 2004b; Hare 2009). Some countries have experiences with removing ATMs from gambling locations. Evaluative studies have shown that the policy reduces gambling intensity among high-risk gamblers (Thomas et al. 2013), but that the effect may be transient (Harrigan et al. 2010).

Cashless transactions, such as playing EGMs directly with a bank or credit card, smart cards or mobile phone, as well as e-banks, wireless technologies, instant loans, and online gambling make access to additional funds even easier (KPMG Consulting 2002; Lähteenmaa and Strand 2008). A narrow policy focus on restricting ATMs or EFTPOS terminals could pave the way for other means of accessing funds depending on the venue and type of EGM.

Gambling on credit has been banned in many jurisdictions across Canada, Europe, and Australia. In the United States house credit is common (Williams et al. 2012b). Although house credit does provide easy access to funds for those with problems, there is no evidence concerning whether banning house credit would work to reduce excessive gambling. It is likely that players would adjust to such regulations, but the reduced availability of funds is likely to have an effect.

Regulating industry strategies as policy levers

A growing body of research is available on the effects of regulating marketing, game features, and venue characteristics as policy measures. In general, each measure has only a small individual impact in isolation, but they do have potential effects in combination. Thus regulations on only one or two characteristics are unlikely to have significant population level impacts.

Marketing regulations and anti-gambling campaigns

Evidence suggests that regulating advertisement for online gambling may be a good policy choice. A European study (Planzer et al. 2014) found that regulations on the advertisement of land-based gambling do not have an impact on problem gambling levels, but strict regulations on online gambling advertisement are statistically connected to lower levels of gambling problems. Vulnerable groups are responsive to marketing, but it is difficult to exclude them from non-personalized campaigns.

Anti-gambling publicity includes warnings in venues and on products but also "public service announcements" in the mass media. A review found that such campaigns are relatively common but few people actually notice or remember them (see Williams et al. 2012b). Evidence from related fields has similarly shown that while changes in knowledge and attitudes may occur, changes in behavior are less common. According to one study, anti-gambling advertisements may even elicit a positive overall image of gambling (Lemarié 2012).

Efforts targeted at high-risk groups appear to be more effective when they encourage problem gamblers to seek help (Jackson et al. 2002). Awareness programmes targeting children and adolescents have also shown promising results. A systematic review of available evaluations shows that school-based education programmes (Breen et al. 2017) reduce cognitive misconceptions about gambling, but the changes decrease over time and do not always translate to behavioral changes. More comprehensive programs with booster sessions performed better. Teaching school children mathematical basics of randomness and probability were also better strategies than promoting ideas of gambling as a harmful activity.

Jackpots, return rates, and bet sizes

Some studies suggest that restricting the size or availability of jackpots reduces the impulse to play by problem gamblers, but it is likely to lower the interest by other players as well. Lowering jackpots is therefore unlikely to target heavy users specifically, but its effect is not limited to moderate or infrequent players either (Crewe-Brown et al. 2014; Williams et al. 2012b).

The return rates (RTP ratios) are not readily known to customers, and other factors determine their willingness to participate. Lotteries usually have big jackpots but very low return rates, yet they are attractive to large numbers of participants. RTP ratios are most problematic around a range of 75% to 92%.

Regulating jackpot size and return rates in the public interest should not be considered only by the effects on problem gambling; it also increases transparency and provides objective information on realistic winning chances, especially in cases where fallacious hopes are an important motivation to play.

The evidence on bet size is inconclusive. The most lucrative Australian EGMs have a high average bet size (Livingstone and Woolley 2008), and high bets intensify the arousal. In many European jurisdictions, machines with large maximum bets and jackpots are located in restricted gambling venues such as casinos, while low-stake gambling machines are permitted in convenience locations. On the other hand, very small bet sizes are commonly used by operators to keep players "in the zone" and maintain their interest in spending on games. In some cases reduced bet sizes have increased participation. To achieve intended effects, the reduction of maximum bets should be substantial, and possibilities for circumvention should be blocked. Policy on bet size should therefore not be limited only to particular games and they should be coupled with personal identity checks.

Many countries apply restrictions on total amount of losses rather than bet sizes per game run. In the Netherlands, for example, losses in non-casino EGMs are limited to 40 EUR an hour, whereas losses in casino EGMs are unlimited (Williams et al. 2012b). In many countries maximum total bet per hour, day, week or month is limited in online games.

Access to cash and form of pay-outs

Policy experiences with removing note acceptors and limiting access to credit have shown promising results. Credits and losses on the game should be shown in real rather than abstract money, whereas complicating the re-use of the winnings in gambling, for instance by payouts in cashable checks or credit notes rather than immediate cash payments, would be an effective harm minimization tactic (Rodda and Cowie 2005; McMillen and Pitt 2005). Paying winnings by check or vouchers instead of cash, and frequent mandatory pay-outs, might effectively break the illusion of winning (Schellinck and Schrans 2002).

Speed, sound, and visual effects of the games

Speed reductions can have an impact if they are sufficiently large and consistently implemented. An Australian policy experiment (Blaszczynski et al. 2001) did not find any significant difference in money or time spent playing between individuals who played EGMs with a 3.5 second event frequency and those playing with a five second event frequency. However, a Canadian laboratory study (Ladouceur and Sévigny 2006) found that reducing the EGM event frequency from five to 15 seconds did reduce play. Other evidence indicates that reducing speed may reduce gambling among at-risk gamblers (Mentzoni et al. 2012). Mandatory pay-outs at regular intervals introduce useful breaks to the spell that may otherwise lead to over-spending.

Sound and visual effects of the games, combined with encouragement of faulty cognitions (bet lines, stop buttons, practice sites), frequent small wins, near misses, and LDWs, have an impact on game intensity and they have a role in masking the real chances of winning. Elements that influence players' immersion in the play, including game themes and modalities of player-player or player-machine interactions, are obvious targets of regulation in the public interest, but they involve difficulties that are similar to regulations of marketing.

Venue designs

Modifications on venue design may help gamblers remain in better control of their play and prevent problems before they escalate. Such modifications are not costly, and some restrictions have already been implemented in many jurisdictions.

Smoking and alcohol use in gambling venues should be prohibited or discouraged. Regulating these behaviors has potential benefits extending beyond the aim of reducing the intent to play and its intensity. Problem gambling is associated with smoking and drinking, and simultaneous access to all of these addictive behaviors reinforces them mutually. Some inducements may mislead customers to believe that they have free bonuses without realizing that they are covering the cost with their gambling losses.

There is no direct evidence on the effectiveness of policy interventions in the case of some other venue characteristics, but practical experience of operators suggests that they do reinforce gambling behavior and their regulation is therefore likely to have an impact. These include the acoustic ambience of gaming environments, their spatial design, and time awareness related to lighting. Immersive casino designs typically combine characteristics of cubicles and open space for different games in ways that may encourage problematic gambling. Online gambling environments often resemble the kinds of recreational or social gaming that are without monetary risks.

Conclusion

Game features and environment characteristics that increase game intensity and players' immersion are relatively well known: speed, near wins and frequent small wins, visual and auditory stimuli, features that prompt competence illusions, and in some cases high jackpots are such game features. Social responsibility tools, such as AsTERiG or GamGard, are already used to evaluate the risks of games based on a variety of such parameters (Meyer et al. 2010). Access to money, time awareness features, inducements, smoking and drinking, and venue design characteristics are known to influence gambling intensity and immersion. Some research suggests that is affected by the regulation of these features and amenities.

Sometimes it is difficult to distinguish research that aims to identify potential risk parameters of games and environments from studies that actually serve the purpose of attracting different types of potential gamblers. Research on policy levers typically measures problem gambling or its intensity as the target variable, often in terms of population effects or risk factors related to game features or venue characteristics. It should be kept in mind that industry strategies vary depending on the context. When markets are expanding, attracting new customers before competitors do is probably a priority. In markets approaching a saturation level, increasing the intensity of play is more relevant, but this, too, can be achieved either by encouraging customers to stay "in the zone" or to spend what they can as fast as possible. It is important to maintain a constant flow of newly introduced gamblers to replace heavy users who can no longer afford to play or have recovered from the habit. Industry strategies are always a mix of these aims.

Policy measures in the public interest have the potential to prevent gambling-related problems significantly, but their targets should be considered in view of the context. In some circumstances it is important to prevent abusive marketing practices, game features, and venue designs. The line is thin between abusiveness and fair methods of selling dreams and imaginary, non-tangible experiences. Considerations of how this line should be drawn must, in the public interest, give sufficient weight to the fact that a significant part of the business serves vulnerable sub-populations that are at risk of causing irreparable harm to themselves, to their families and other people affected, and to society at large. A large part of those being initiated to gambling do not understand the risks and the real chances of winning. Transparency and honesty, however difficult to affirm, should in all cases have priority over monetary interests, public or private.

Given the heavy concentration of consumption in high-risk groups, successful preventive methods tend to cut down the volume of spending, profits and the surplus. Reducing gambling problems without reducing revenue is thus not a realistic goal. Efforts directed mostly to keep down problematic gambling without affecting the total volume of the trade are successful only in limited cases, for example, preventing underage gambling, avoiding game offers targeted only to small minorities of very heavy users, and keeping venue locations away from areas populated by vulnerable groups.

Policy measures must be consistent and sufficiently comprehensive in order to be effective. Policymakers can determine the kind of game, venue, and marketing strategies gambling providers can offer. Gambling providers should be mandated to prove that a product, an advertisement or a venue is safe *before* it is launched to players.

Chapter 9

Pre-commitment and interventions in risk behavior

The essence of gambling is that outcomes of game runs are fortuitous and vary a great deal from loss of the wager to gains that amount to multiple times its value. On average, the "house"—the operator of the game—always wins, but the individual might also be inclined to believe that the time has come to "beat the odds". The hope for the winning line and excitement about the result are the key factors that seduce players, some occasionally and others habitually, to continue the game beyond their resources in time and especially money.

The impulse to continue can be restrained by pre-commitments that set an advance limit to amounts of time and money to be spent on the game. Once reached, the limits cannot be exceeded without a new decision to continue, sometimes requiring a time break or other impediments to follow the impulse. Pre-commitments are the most commonly applied strategy to prevent excessive gambling, one that is frequently included in responsible gambling policies offered by the industry (Williams et al. 2012b).

Another common component of "responsible gambling policies" that may be required of or offered by the industry is intervention in high-risk behavior by an individual gambler. Such interventions can be undertaken by gambling staff, or interventions can occur in an automated way to initiate or supervise pre-commitments and to encourage help-seeking.

Whether in the form of a pre-commitment chosen by the gambler or a warning sign or personal intervention by others in the case of high-risk behavior, the measures considered in this chapter focus on the behavior of the gambler as an individual. This tends to make such measures more acceptable, at least in principle, to gambling providers: the focus of the measure is on deficiencies or worries of the individual gambler, and not on characteristics of the services being sold by the provider. The measures thus fit the industry's preferred framing of gambling problems in terms of defective individuals rather than anything about the activity in general.

Pre-commitments and interventions can be implemented in several ways. First, pre-commitment can be mandatory or voluntary. Measures can either be put in place for all gamblers, or they can be voluntarily implemented at the player's own discretion.

Second, pre-commitment can be based on legislative interventions or as part of operators' own corporate social responsibility (CSR) measures. Monopolistic operators use CSR to distinguish themselves as a responsible alternative to private competition, while online gambling companies have joined together to set voluntary industry standards such as the e-Commerce and Online Gaming Regulation and Assurance Agency (eCOGRA) and the Interactive Gaming Council (IGC). Some countries require CSR measures from operators as a condition of a license.

Third, pre-commitment can be based on self-assessment or play-assessment. Self-assessment refers to players' own assessment of their behavior, and includes measures of self-control by limit-setting, self-evaluations, and self-exclusion. Play-assessment is based on observed gambling behavior of an individual. This can be accomplished either through automated algorithms based on player data or through staff interventions. Play-assessment is particularly well suited for online gambling, as all gambling activity is recorded. Smart card technology allows similar measures in land-based venues.

The majority of pre-commitment tools in use today are voluntary and based on self-assessment. The approach emphasizes individual autonomy and understands *responsible gambling* as the responsibility of the individual, rather than that of the industry or the government (Schüll 2012).

Warning signs

Some games and venues incorporate warning signs to encourage player responsibility and auto-regulation. The content of warnings ranges from information on the risks and the odds of the game, to encouraging gamblers to stay within affordable limits. Advertising for help services is often included (Monaghan and Blaszczynski 2010a). The approach is in line with the "informed choice" framework that has been argued to reflect the interests of the gambling industry rather than actual advances in consumer protection (McGowan 2001).

Studies have shown that information may increase problem awareness but has little impact on gambling intensity (see Monaghan and Blaszczynski 2010b for a review). A comparative study reported no difference in gambling behavior between jurisdictions that have and have not introduced warning labels on lottery products (McGowan 2001). A survey of Australian gamblers (n = 954) has shown that while players do notice the warnings, only a small minority report that they have any impact on gambling behavior, and a majority are sceptical of their effectiveness in general (Hing 2003). A laboratory experiment by Lambos and Delfabbro (2007) found that gamblers are typically already aware of the risks of gambling, but this knowledge does not necessarily translate into actions.

More promising results have been obtained regarding dynamic warnings. A study by Monaghan and Blaszczynski (2007) noted that 83% of EGM players recalled the content of dynamic pop-up warnings, while only 15% of the same participants recalled the content of static warning signs. A follow-up study (Monaghan and Blaszczynski 2010b) showed that pop-ups had a more significant impact on gambling thoughts and behavior than static signs. A UK study (Auer et al. 2014) used tracking data of 200,000 online gamblers, and reported that after viewing a pop-up message, nine times more gamblers stopped their session compared to those who had not seen the message.

A Canadian policy experiment implemented a pop-up warning on EGMs after 60 minutes of continuous play. An evaluation of the intervention (Schellinck and Schrans 2002) showed a significant reduction in duration and expenditure among the participants (n = 163). A follow-up study found that pop-up messages 30 minutes after continuous play did not improve the results significantly in comparison to the 60-minute interval (Schrans et al. 2004).

In addition to the type of warning messages, the content of these messages has an impact. Personalized information on pop-ups appears to be more efficient than generic pop-up messages. A recent Australian study conducted at EGM venues (Gainsbury et al. 2015) showed gamblers (n = 667) a series of dynamic warning messages. Participants then completed a questionnaire on how well they recalled the messages and what their impact had been. Results showed that participants recalled messages that encouraged self-assessment, such as "Have you spent more than you can afford?" better than messages containing general information such as "Set your limits. Play within it." Messages that discussed money had the greatest impact on reducing gambling. Monetary reminders were also found effective in a Canadian laboratory study (Stewart and Wohl 2013) in which participants (n = 59) who received a pop-up note on their spending were significantly more likely to adhere to monetary limits than the control group.

A UK study (Auer and Griffiths 2014) used online tracking data to investigate behavioral changes in 279 online gamblers who had signed up for a voluntary personalized feedback on their gambling. Results showed that those who had signed up for the service had reduced the amount and time spent gambling in comparison to the control group (n = 65,432). A more comprehensive implementation combined with player tracking is likely to be the best policy option regarding warnings.

Limit-setting in online environments

Limit-setting is particularly easy to implement online. The Australian Productivity Commission (2010) has recommended a mandatory limit-setting system as one of the most pressing measures to enhance safe online gambling.

Limit-setting tools are available on most gambling websites, but their implementation varies (Lucar et al. 2013). Most sites offer a voluntary option to set limits. Some limits are fixed and operator-imposed, others are mandatory but gamblers are required to fix for themselves the amount of time to be spent, and money either to be spent on purchases or losses. For example, the Austrian Win2Day website has a weekly deposit limit of about 800 EUR. The Finnish state monopoly has a mandatory single player account with a maximum deposit of 20,000 EUR, and a daily maximum loss limit of 1,000 EUR per day or 2,000 EUR per month for fast internet games. The Norwegian monopoly Norsk Tipping sets a personal monthly loss limit at 20,000 NOK (about 2,200 EUR) (Lucar et al. 2013). The New Zealand online lottery limits ticket purchases to 150 NZD a week and 300 NZD (about 200 EUR) a month (Williams et al. 2012b).

There is a growing body of evidence on the effectiveness of online limiting tools. Online gamblers generally accept monetary limits and find them useful (Griffiths et al. 2009b). However, use of voluntary tools remains low. A study based on a sample of 100,000 online gamblers on the Austrian Win2day website reported that only 5% had set some voluntary time or money limits (Auer and Griffiths 2013a). Another study (Nelson et al. 2008) used registry data of 47,000 players on the Austrian Bwin online gambling website. Results showed that only 1% of players had activated the limit-setting feature.

Another study making use of the same Bwin data (Broda et al. 2008) found that the maximum limits proposed by operators are excessively high, for example 100,000 EUR a week. Consequently, only 0.03% of players had ever tried to exceed the limit.

Nevertheless, if it is properly implemented, limit-setting can have positive outcomes by encouraging gamblers to play moderately. Nelson et al. (2008) found that self-limited players experienced declines in amounts wagered and in the frequency of wagers. Ten percent of self-limiters also stopped gambling at the Bwin website after setting limits, but we do not know if they moved to other sites or reduced their total amount spent on gambling.

There is some evidence that limits may be most effective for those who already play excessively or intensely. The study based on the Win2day data (Auer and Griffiths 2013a) found that after setting voluntary limits, the most intense players had significantly reduced money or time spent gambling. It is nevertheless possible that these players simply migrated to another website. Research on the voluntary limit-setting tool PlayScan available on the Swedish governmentally operated Svenska Spel's online poker site found evidence of this kind of evasion; 30% of all players who reached their monetary limits on the site gambled on other sites (Stymne 2008). While this may be a substantial proportion, this also means that a significant majority (70%) did not gamble on other sites, which indicates that the monetary limits worked for some players.

Voluntary limit-setting in online environments can have an impact on individual behavior, but their population-level effect remains marginal. It is probable that a mandatory limit-setting system with reasonable maximum limits would yield better results.

Limit-setting in land-based gambling

Limit-setting has been technically more difficult in land-based venues, but it is not impossible. Smart card technology in EGMs has been tested in a number of jurisdictions across Australia, Canada, and Europe (Williams et al. 2012b). The Netherlands and Finland have introduced visitation limits to casinos as an alternative to a total self-exclusion. A few US states have also tested spending limits on riverboat casino cruises, but these programs have been discontinued to better compete with neighbouring states (Williams et al. 2012b).

Smart cards have been used in gambling as loyalty cards, but the same technology can be programmed into pre-commitment tools. Players insert cards into gambling machines to keep track of their play and to set spending and/or time limits. Mandatory systems require all players to set limits, whereas voluntary schemes do not impose limits but provide an opportunity to do so. In hybrid systems, pre-commitment is only required for high intensity machines (Ladouceur et al. 2012).

A critical review of existing card-based pre-commitment systems (Ladouceur et al. 2012) concludes that voluntary pre-commitment systems are not attractive to players. When cards are voluntary, user rates remain low. A trial conducted in Queensland (Schottler Consulting 2009) with a "SimPlay" option added to existing loyalty cards showed that only 2% of venue members signed up for the feature.

The best researched policy experiment with smart cards comes from Nova Scotia. The Canadian province introduced a player tracking card called My-Play in 2010 and made it mandatory in 2012. The preparation for this reform started in 2005 with a first trial study (Omnifacts Bristol Research 2005). In this study, participants were not required to use the card, but were encouraged to do so. Players were also allowed to choose what kind of limits they wanted to use. Results showed that 45% of players used the card every time they played. A second trial (Omnifacts Bristol Research 2007) made the card mandatory, but players could still choose which features to use. Only 17% of players set some kind of a limit.

Another problem with voluntary cards is that players may simply continue gambling without them after reaching a pre-set limit. The first Nova Scotia trial (Omnifacts Bristol Research 2005) found that 68% of card adopters reached a limit during the trial, but 44% of these players reported having continued playing without the card. This was particularly the case with participants with high problem gambling scores. Furthermore, players have reported that there is some social stigma associated with the use of a voluntary card and that pop-up warnings or beeping sounds reinforce this problem (Schellinck and Schrans 2010).

A mandatory card is likely to have a more significant impact. Studies have shown that players who have adopted smart cards report that it encourages them to gamble more responsibly and to think about spending (Schottler Consulting 2010, 2009; Omnifacts Bristol Research 2005). Card adopters have also reduced their gambling intensity. In the second Nova Scotia trial (Omnifacts Bristol Research 2007), card data showed that 63% of card users (n = 137) reduced their gambling expenditure, while 72% decreased the time spent gambling. In South Australia, card users decreased their spending by 32% in comparison to a control group after the introduction of a limit-setting feature in a popular loyalty card (Schottler Consulting 2010).

Other studies have shown less promising results. In the Queensland study (Schottler Consulting 2009), 79% of respondents reported that smart cards had no impact on expenditure. A pre- and post-use comparison among card adopters (n = 122) in Nova Scotia (Schellinck and Schrans 2007) also found that while these individuals had significantly reduced their spending on gambling, they had increased the length of play sessions. There was also no change in terms of frequency of play per month, suggesting that the card did not end up having the expected impact on gambling.

The final study conducted for the Nova Scotia trials (Schellinck and Schrans 2010) concluded that smart cards should be mandatory to be fully effective. Unfortunately, there have been no reliable studies on policy experiments with mandatory smart cards. The Norwegian case is the most comprehensive example of a full pre-commitment system available today.

Mandatory player cards were introduced in Norwegian EGMs, sports betting, and online gambling in 2009. Limits are defined by the operator, and cannot exceed 600 NOK (about 65 EUR) per day or 2,500 NOK (about 270 EUR) per month (Leino et al. 2015). The policy reform also included a complete redesign of EGMs by introducing the Multix terminal (see Figure 9.1). In addition to various limit-setting options, the machine implements many of the interface-based restrictions described in Chapter 8, including limiting speed, and displaying the credit balance in NOK. There are currently no conclusive studies available on the effects of the policy reform. The levels of problem gambling did rise in Norway to 4.4% in the 2010 prevalence study, in comparison to 3.1% and 3.6% in 2008 and 2009 respectively, but declined later to a level below the initial rate (Rossow and Hansen 2016). However, as observed in Chapter 4, prevalence estimates from population studies are uncertain.

Introduction of mandatory smart cards in other jurisdictions has seen a considerable decline in EGM revenue. The mandatory smart card in Nova Scotia was discontinued in 2014 after a drop of 25% in EGM revenue for the province

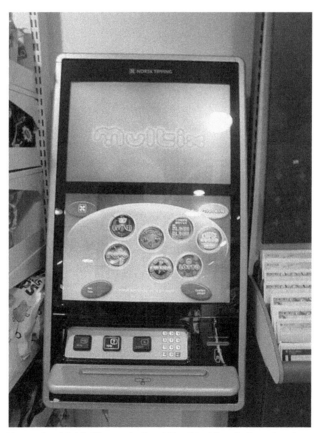

Fig 9.1 A Norwegian Multix Electronic Gambling Machine designed to decrease problem
Photograph by Sjurmh, distributed under a CC BY-SA 3.0 license.

between 2012 and 2014. Within weeks of removing the card, revenue had again increased by about 11%. In Sweden, a 25% decline in EGM revenue was also registered in 2014 following a mandatory player card system, although competition from online gambling may also partially explain the drop in revenue (Lotteriinspektionen 2015). This indicates that mandatory player cards can have a significant impact on gambler behavior, but consequently the turnover of the operators is likely to fall as a consequence.

Self-exclusion and other exclusion policies

Self-exclusion programs provide a temporary break from gambling by allowing individuals to voluntarily ban themselves from entering one or multiple gaming venues. In case of breaches, the ban is sometimes enforced by penalties for the self-excluded gamblers, but rarely for providers. In some jurisdictions, like New Zealand, venues are subject to significant fines for allowing self-excluded gamblers to gamble on their premises. However, evidence to support the efficacy of this approach is not extensive (Gainsbury 2014). Recent reports indicate that the Auckland casino will introduce facial recognition software for the purpose of enforcing self-exclusion (Fisher 2013).

Bans vary in duration and design. In most jurisdictions, including North America and Australia, exclusion bans are strictly voluntary (South Australian Centre for Economic Studies 2003; Thompson 2010). In some countries, such as Singapore, family members may initiate the ban, while in others, casino staff may impose exclusions or visitation limitations. In countries like Switzerland, the Netherlands and South Korea, exclusion programs are interlinked with employee education and a monitoring system of gamblers' behavior (Thompson 2010; Kingma 2015).

Self-exclusions are the predominant harm reduction strategy used by the gambling industry. It is an extreme form of pre-commitment. The effectiveness of self-exclusion programs can be measured in three ways: by their utilization rate, by the percentage of self-excluded patrons who do not re-enter casinos during the contracted period of exclusion, and by the impact self-exclusion policies have on overall gambling participation. Based on these yardsticks, self-exclusion policies do not seem to be very effective in many jurisdictions (Williams et al. 2012b). According to a questionnaire study (Responsible Gambling Council 2006), problem gamblers also consider self-exclusions to be one of the least effective tools to control their gambling.

Relatively few gamblers choose to self-exclude. A population survey from Victoria showed that only 0.06% of the adult population had excluded themselves from gambling venues, although 1% of the same population had been identified as problem gamblers (see Brown 2010). In Canada, an estimated 0.6% to 7% of problem gamblers self-exclude (Williams 2012b). European jurisdictions have reported somewhat higher use rates. In the Netherlands, a study of 450 regular gamblers (De Bruin et al. 2006) showed that 13% had an entry limitation.

There is evidence that customers manage to enter casinos despite a pre-set self-exclusion. The number of breaches is larger in jurisdictions without centralized registers and entrance controls. A Québec study found that 36% of self-excluders interviewed (n = 220) returned to the casino during the self-exclusion period (Ladouceur et al. 2000). A Nova Scotia study showed that 33% of surveyed self-excluders (n = 76) breached the ban, and that 70% of these breaches went undetected (Responsible Gambling Council 2008). Breaches are also common in Australia, but detection rates have been better (Croucher et al. 2006). In European and some Asian jurisdictions, mandatory identity checks at casino entrances effectively prevent breaches and make self-exclusion programs more viable (Lhommeau 2015; Thompson 2010; De Bruin et al. 2006). In Germany, for example, self-exclusions are assembled into one register for banned casino players, sport-bettors, and instant-lottery gamblers (Meyer and Bachmann 2011). Review studies by Williams et al. (2012b) and Gainsbury (2014) acknowledge effective identification of customers to be a major issue in the enforcement of self-exclusion agreements between gamblers and venues.

When self-exclusions are thoroughly enforced, they have the potential to reduce gambling intensity and to improve self-control. Preliminary evidence suggests that self-exclusion can be effective in online environments, where identification is generally required (Hayer and Meyer 2011b). Evidence from New South Wales shows that self-excluders (n = 135) had reduced gambling expenditure by half (Croucher et al. 2006). A longitudinal Canadian study (Ladouceur et al. 2007) with 161 self-excluders from Québec showed that the urge to gamble was significantly reduced during the 6, 12, 18, and 24-month follow-ups and players rated their sense of control over their gambling higher. However, this study also demonstrated that about half of those in the cohort had breached their self-exclusion regularly and returned to a casino, and 67% of the original cohort left the study during its course (Livingstone et al. 2014).

Other research has suggested that self-excluders may rebound after an initial decline in gambling activity, and many return to their previous levels (Hayer and Meyer 2011a; De Bruin et al. 2001). Williams et al. (2012b) suggest that self-exclusion can start a natural path to recovery but needs support from other forms of treatment. This can be accomplished by providing more services, reducing barriers to program entry (Gainsbury 2014; Blaszczynski et al. 2007), and by more significant provider involvement.

Bans on cheaters and criminals that aim at protecting the casino's interests are enforced to a much higher degree than voluntary self-exclusion (Kingma 2015), and show that an effective control is possible.

Staff training and interventions

In most jurisdictions, casino and gambling venue staff receive some training to identify and deal with problem gamblers, and to direct them to treatment and other help. Holland Casinos in the Netherlands was the first to provide an intensive training and education program for employees, as early as the late 1980s. Today, staff training is part of the American Gaming Association's Code of Conduct for Responsible Gaming, the European Casino Association's Code of Conduct, and the World Lotteries Association Code of Conduct.

Staff training is a relatively useful tool to identify problem gambling. Most training programs introduce initiation of pre-commitment strategies and means to supervise them. Field tests (Delfabbro et al. 2012; Haefeli et al. 2011) have shown that staff members are mostly able to identify a problem gambler correctly. Interview studies also indicate that staff members consider training to be useful (LaPlante et al. 2012; Dufour et al. 2010). Some studies have reported proactive interventions by staff members after receiving training, although the changes were not fully maintained at a follow-up (Ladouceur et al. 2004; Dufour et al. 2010). This suggests that staff training programs should take place at regular intervals to preserve their impact. There is also some evidence that training and interventions may be effective in online environments (Häfeli et al. 2011).

Nevertheless, quantitative evidence has shown that the effect of staff interventions may be insignificant at a population level. Switzerland has introduced a program in which casino employees are obliged to approach customers who meet the criteria of a problem gambler checklist. Evaluations of this program have shown that only 0.01% of all customers, and 16.6% of prospective self-excluders had ever been contacted. Furthermore, in 80–90% of these cases, interventions consisted of only a brief discussion, without further action taken (Haefeli and Lischer 2010; Williams et al. 2012b). No evidence is available supporting the effectiveness of these interventions.

One reason for the ineffectiveness of staff interventions has been lax implementation (Rintoul et al. 2017). Furthermore, training does not always address the right problems. Staff training helps in identifying problem gamblers, but does not give adequate guidance on how to intervene (Delfabbro et al. 2007). Interview studies have shown that staff can be reluctant to approach probable problem gamblers because they fear getting in trouble with their manager or with the customers

(Hing and Nuske 2011; 2012). Based on this evidence, staff training should involve methods and techniques to help staff become more confident in approaching potential problem gamblers, such as role playing exercises that are already in use in Switzerland.

Automated interventions

In addition to staff interventions, automated tools based on play assessment (tracking) can be used to identify problem gambling patterns and to intervene before problems escalate. Automated tools are particularly useful in online environments, in which technological software can be used to track gambling behavior (e.g., PlayScan, Bet Buddy, Mentor) (Lucar et al. 2013).

The PlayScan tool gives feedback to players on risk levels of their activity, and alerts the player of status changes. In addition, PlayScan centralizes limit-setting, gambling profiles, and the possibility to self-exclude in one place. The tool is used by several governmentally-operated gambling sites in Europe, and is also available on Swedish EGMs. Research has shown that players regard PlayScan as useful (Griffiths et al. 2009b), but user rates remain low if it is voluntary. A questionnaire study with Swedish website clientele (n = 2,348) (Griffiths et al. 2009b) found that 26% had used PlayScan. Another Swedish study (Forsström et al. 2016) showed that user rates decline over time.

Like limit-setting tools, play assessment tools appear to only reach their full potential if mandatory. According to behavioral tracking data (n = 779), non-problem and at-risk gamblers who had adopted PlayScan reduced the intensity of their gambling, but players most at risk did not show significant reductions in gambling (Wood and Wohl 2015). If the tool is not mandatory, cautious gamblers may be more likely to use it and the measured effects may only show a difference between cautious and risk-taking players, rather than reflecting the actual effectiveness of the feedback function.

In land-based venues, tracking data from player cards can be used to create automated interventions. In New Zealand, reward card data is used to track EGM expenditure and the frequency of visits to the casino. The most intense players can be excluded based on this information. Automated interventions can also be based on visitation data when identification is required at casino entrance. In countries such as the Netherlands and Austria, casinos record and track the entries of each customer. In the case of a significant increase in visits or a high number of visits over time, the system alerts personnel to intervene or to impose a short ban from the venue (Williams et al. 2012b). In the Netherlands, a large number of interventions take place every year, but research has shown that 60% of possible problem gamblers have still never been approached by staff (Kingma 2015). This is likely to be related to the problems with staff interventions as already described, rather than to the ineffectiveness of the automated tool.

When identity controls are not in use in casinos, facial recognition software may be a solution to prevent self-excluded problem gamblers from entering the venue. In Saskatchewan, a system called iCare combines facial recognition with a tracking card to identify problem gamblers (Williams et al. 2012b). The iCare is a predictive algorithm that detects problem behavior and communicates it to the casino management. Marketing to the player can be frozen and the player may be denied entry to the venue. Combined with observations of trained employees, the system identified 95% of problem gamblers correctly (Schüll 2012). However, there is no data available on whether the system actually contributes to changing problematic gambling patterns.

Conclusions

In this chapter, we have discussed research evidence on pre-commitment tools and other interventions designed to help individual players to better control their gambling. The gambling industry has responsibilities, either self-imposed or mandated by law and other regulations, to protect players from problem gambling, but also a financial interest in gambling revenues. These responsibilities and financial interests partly coincide. Excessive gambling can be harmful for the business as an image problem, as well as a nuisance in the venue, leading to rapid insolvency of regulars, and spoiling the appeal for new gamblers. On the other hand, heavy users contribute a substantial share of the operators' revenue, and limits to their spending may reduce profits. The balance may be difficult to find.

The most common solution is to adopt measures that tend to be the least effective. These include static warnings and measures based on self-assessment that mostly serve to exhibit the operators' corporate social responsibility (CSR). When more effective tools such as player tracking and limit-setting are implemented, they are often done in such a "perfunctory fashion as to virtually ensure lack of impact" (Williams et al. 2012b: 81).

The studies reviewed in this chapter indicate that some pre-commitment strategies can be effective if properly managed. Such programs are not costly or difficult to implement. Online gambling sites already track players' activity, and the data can easily be used to protect consumers. Land-based gambling venues renew their EGMs regularly to keep up gambler interest (Woolley & Livingstone 2010), and card-readers can easily be integrated in the new machines without the need to carry out costly upgrades on the machines currently operating (Australian Productivity Commission 2010).

The discussion in this chapter has shown that pre-commitment effectiveness can be improved in four different ways. First, the measures should be personalized. Evidence shows that static warning signs have as little effect in this area as in other lifestyle-related risk issues. Warnings should be dynamic and combined with personalized information collected through player tracking.

Second, pre-commitment tools should be mandatory and non-selective. Voluntary, self-imposed pre-commitment strategies have the potential to be effective, but user rates remain low. This is particularly true of limit-setting in online environments, smart card technology in EGMs, and PlayScan-type tools where individual gambling behavior can be tracked. Efficient techniques to reduce harm are available but if they are designed to target only high-risk or problem gamblers they may well have adverse stigma effects. Limits should be sufficently low to deter excessive spenders, who frequently have low incomes.

Third, providers have to take significant responsibility for the implementation of any pre-commitment strategy. *Responsible gambling* should refer not only to the responsibility of players, but include providers' responsibility for product safety, consumer protection and harm avoidance (Livingstone and Adams 2011).

Gambling providers should complement self-exclusion policies with resources for the self-excluded, and there should also be legal action against providers who fail to respect the self-exclusion contract. Staff training should be repeated at regular intervals, covering not only how to detect problem gamblers, but also how to remove barriers for staff to intervene effectively and offer assistance. Automated detection should always lead to an intervention, not just at the operator's discretion. Identification of problem gamblers is not enough; it is also important to consider what happens next. Finally, providers need to be involved in designing reasonable limit-setting options. Online providers in particular have a lot of room in which to move. Tracking allows many responsible gambling initiatives to work best on the internet (Monaghan 2008). Tracking-based tools to protect players should be a condition of licensing.

A fourth way to improve pre-commitment programs is to expand them in new directions. Some suggestions have included a license to gamble (Goss and Morse 2009), but also heavy restrictions on what types of games operators are actually allowed to provide and under what conditions. Sound ethical principles should be applied in considering to what population segments games are offered, and economic consequences for spenders as well as for beneficiaries should be included in these. This is an area where more research is most urgently needed.

Problems in the implementation of pre-commitment tools reduce their overall population-level effect. The more limited the implementation of a pre-commitment tool, the more limited is its impact (Williams et al. 2012b). In conclusion, pre-commitment has the potential to work if purchasing or loss limits are set at reasonable levels, but its implementation has to be connected to actual risk behavior, to be mandatory, to be combined with other preventive measures, and to include not only the commitment of players, but also of legislators and providers.

Chapter 10

Gambling control regimes

Gambling regulation by governments is undertaken for four reasons. First, gambling involves an excess of revenue over the cost of providing the service, and sharing in this is attractive to governments. Second, governments wish to prevent fraud, crime, and corruption attracted by money flows that will be intractable if left outside a regulated market. Third, regulation often aims to lower the risk of harm and to provide consumer protection. Finally, as shown in Chapter 2, moral concerns, have, at least historically, played a part in regulation; highly regulated gambling regimes usually originated as an alternative to a prior prohibition. These aims are sometimes contradictory. Fiscal interests may not be best served by policies aimed at limiting harm and at preventing malpractices. Governments inevitably face conflicts of interest between such aims.

Regulation can be conducted in several organizational forms and is located in different branches of government in different countries. Also international agreements and bodies are involved in gambling regulation.

This chapter describes the types of regulation in different jurisdictions and assesses relative strengths and weaknesses in implementing policies to reduce harm from gambling, their efficiency in collecting money for public use, their capacity to maintain the integrity of games, and their ability to prevent fraud and crime related to addiction. Comparative research in this area is scarce, but case studies can shed light on the different ways in which regulations can be put in place.

Regimes

Whenever the state exerts control over the gambling market there are four main alternatives: 1) prohibition; 2) public monopolies, often but not always operated and owned by states; 3) licensing; and 4) the free market. The primary aim of this chapter is to focus on regulatory control regimes in categories 2) and 3). A truly free market has no regulations, and is rare in modern societies for any commercial commodity or activity. Gambling policies in most countries aim to limit the unregulated market in favor of the regulated one, either to prevent harm or for financial reasons. Prohibitions are also rare and usually cover only some forms of gambling.

A government can run a gambling enterprise itself, as a public body. The justification for this choice is often that the gambling provision will then be run in the public interest, with considerations of private profit not entering into market decisions. Such a justification, for instance, has been the primary rationale for government gambling monopolies in the Nordic countries.

Such a government-run enterprise is often termed a "monopoly" in current parlance even when in reality it is not one, because the market includes competing gambling providers (whether from other jurisdictions or in terms of other providers the government has licensed). Thus a government-run lottery may face competition from lotteries run by charities, private companies or those which the government itself has licensed.

In most modern states, gambling is subject to special legislation that defines the terms and conditions of the activity, normally supervised by one or several government regulatory bodies and controlled by one or several ministries. Licenses are often granted to associations, churches, and charities that channel the proceeds to finance their own activities or good causes they themselves represent. Alternatively, licenses may be made available to private enterprise. The number of licenses allowed is often limited; in a highly profitable industry, this means that the license in itself is often a valuable property.

Limited access to the market reduces the incentive for competition on price, allowing a greater surplus of profit than in a competitive market. In many jurisdictions a license is sold to a single private bidder, with considerable revenue coming to the state, for example the Australian state of Victoria, with its single license for a private casino.

The regime in a jurisdiction may also vary between different forms of gambling. Thus it is quite common for one form of gambling to be monopolized, a second to be licensed, and a third forbidden. Lotteries tend to be government-controlled monopolies, while horse racing and bingo rarely are. Casinos in the United States are private, but in many European countries they are provided by a public operator or a restricted number of licensed private operators closely supervised by the state (Williams et al. 2012b).

Government departments and non-governmental organizations (NGOs) are the most common beneficiaries of the gambling surplus, and therefore important interests in the politics of gambling availability (Rand and Light 2006). In many cases government departments channel the money to earmarked purposes, especially sports, culture, scientific research, education, social services, youth work, medical care, and patient organizations. Business corporations may participate in projects funded from gambling sources. These factors lead to different configurations even in cases where similar regulatory forms are applied, making comparisons between regimes very difficult. However, it is possible to arrive at a series of considerations to be taken into account whenever regulatory regimes are redesigned or reassessed.

Prohibition

Bringing unregulated gambling under government control has been a major justification for the expansion of legal markets.

Some countries have attempted to prohibit online but not land-based gambling. A successful prohibition would have to be coupled with effective restrictions on offshore operators (Gainsbury and Wood 2011). The United States is a good example. The country first tried to impose restrictions on online gambling in 1998 by prosecuting foreign-based suppliers, but with limited success (Paoli 2014). In 2006, the Unlawful Internet Gambling Enforcement Act (UIGEA) introduced payment blocking and the targeting of credit card and other global payment systems instead of direct government control of gambling provision. In 2010 only 0.5% of Americans gambled online (Debaise 2011).

Monopoly regimes

Government-controlled monopolies offer governments the advantages of direct political steering, simple supervisory structure, and efficient transfer of the surplus to government budgets. State gambling monopolies can be found in Canada, Luxembourg, Switzerland, Slovakia, and the Nordic countries, but they cover only a segment of the market. Private gambling monopolies are operated by companies and foundations or associations with exclusive licenses based on competitive tendering or other selection processes (Planzer 2014). For example, in Australia, casino monopoly franchises are granted to private companies based on a bidding process. Joint-ventures refer to industry-government cooperation. This model is common in Canadian casinos. Some countries have chosen to apply the monopoly model to online gambling as well. This has been the case in Sweden, Canada, and Hong Kong. Gambling on unauthorized sites may still continue in these contexts, as governments have not been able to compete fully with offshore options (Gainsbury and Wood 2011; Abovitz 2008).

State lotteries are the most protected national monopolies and important public revenue generators, even in countries with otherwise competitive gambling markets. A cross-national comparative study of 125 state lotteries found that 48% of jurisdictions had licensed a private company to operate a monopoly lottery. Another 48% of jurisdictions had state-owned companies, or ran lotteries directly through a designated ministry or department. In some cases, national lotteries are licensed to non-profit organizations. The majority of countries in Africa, Asia, and South America have contracted their national lotteries to private operators. In Europe and North America, the majority of jurisdictions had government-operated lotteries (Gidluck 2016).

The National Lottery in the UK highlights the role state lotteries have in a free-market context. It is the most popular and most commonly available form of gambling in the country. The National Lottery has provided either the Exchequer (government treasury) or benefitting organizations with over 2.2 billion GBP. It is run on behalf of the government by a privately owned company with its own commercial interests unrelated to the government business it undertakes (Lepper and Creigh-Tyte 2013).

In comparison with other forms of gambling, state lotteries are a cost-efficient vehicle for public revenue collection (McGowan 2001), as they have high tax rates and low return rates. Citizens may equate paying for lottery tickets with helping to support good causes. This hides the fact that revenues from state lotteries are mostly collected from low-income segments of the population, and thus constitute a very regressive form of taxation (Beckert and Lutter 2013). Those in welfare assistance programs participate more often than others in lotteries (Grote and Matheson 2011).

Licensing

Licensing systems vary in their degree of competitiveness and in what kinds of operators are eligible. Some jurisdictions allow a limited number of gambling machines or venues while not restricting the license to a single provider. Only one form of gambling may be covered, or several may be licensed. The market may involve a mixture of state-operated, non-profit, and private market actors.

Licensing has become a popular approach in online environments even in countries with long-established restrictive monopoly systems. Norway allowed offshore gambling operators in 2004. The UK opened its online gambling markets to competition with the 2005 Gambling Act. France and Italy opened their online markets to licensed operators in 2010, followed by Spain in 2011, Denmark in 2012 and Portugal in 2015. The trend is linked to strong economic incentives for governments but also aims to maintain the integrity and social responsibility of online gambing (Gainsbury and Wood 2011).

Licensing can be limited to domestic gambling providers (termed "closed regulation") or also allow operators based elsewhere ("open regulation"; Abovitz 2008).

The United Kingdom is an example of open regulation. Since 2005, operators are required to obtain a license from the Gambling Commission and subject themselves to conditions and monitoring to ensure compliance with licensing requirements. Licensed operators can accept wagers from anywhere in the world (Abovitz 2008). There are approximately 3,000 gambling license holders in the United Kingdom. The UK system has been described as a successful approach, as it has increased employment and tax revenue by capturing a portion of the international online market (Abovitz 2008). It is argued that the regime has been designed to tempt business from the least regulated jurisdictions to a jurisdiction with relatively high standards that will also help online gambling companies gain legitimacy and stability (Beem and Mikler 2011).

France is an example of closed regulation. Since 2010 a government body called ARJEL (Autorité de régulation du jeu en ligne) grants and supervises gambling licenses to online providers with a physical address in France. Only three types of online gambling are allowed: sports betting, horse race betting, and poker, as they are considered less dangerous than games of pure chance. Online lotteries are only provided by a national monopoly. The French system has been described as relatively successful, as it has been able to channel online gambling to licensed websites and increase tax revenue (ARJEL 2015).

Australia has a system similar to France. Australia was one of the first countries to implement online gambling legislation (Gainsbury and Wood 2011), but the Interactive Gambling Act (IGA) of 2001 only allows purchase of lottery tickets and wagering (including sports betting) online. Online casinos and in-play sports betting are excluded, since they are regarded as more dangerous (Abovitz 2008). Australians can still gamble on offshore sites offering games that are not allowed in Australia, but this is not a widespread activity (Victorian Responsible Gambling Foundation 2014; Gainsbury and Wood 2011).

Associations and charities

Associations, charities, and other non-profit organizations can also offer some form of gambling, often in the context of a monopoly or licensing system. Originally these organizations had limited aims: to collect money for public or private uses, but as gambling has become commercialized, the line between non-profits, government monopolies, and private enterprises has become blurred. A comparative study of charity bingos concluded that charity gambling can be both effective and socially just, but the model should not be privileged unconditionally (Bedford et al. 2016). Some Canadian provinces have charity casinos that operate on a much smaller scale than "destination casinos". In 2013, Alberta had 3,448 charity casino licenses. In British Columbia, charity casino licenses are granted for social occasions, and in provinces like Saskatchewan and Manitoba charities can organize so-called "Monte Carlo nights" (Responsible Gambling Council 2015).

Canadian charities also organize larger lotteries such as the Princess Margaret Hospital Lottery and the Heart and Stroke Lottery. In 2011, nearly 17,000 charity lotteries were licensed to operate in Canada. In comparison to government-operated lotteries in Canada, charity lotteries are less efficient in raising revenue, and not always even profitable. This is partly due to marketing expenses because while government-run lotteries are weekly, charity lotteries need to advertise when their draws occur (Thomson and Cheng 2013).

In most Australian states, the private club industry and hotels of bars offer EGM gambling in locations that are formally provided for members, but widely accessible to others. Organizations such as the Returned Services League (aimed to support former or current Australian servicemen and women or their dependents) carry licenses, and many are members of Clubs Australia, an association of 6,500 member organizations offering gambling in Australia. The offer may include only a few slot machines in a golf club-house, but may also be quite extensive and casino-like, particularly in the most populous Australian state, New South Wales, where EGMs have been permitted in such clubs since 1956. Currently clubs have licenses for 70% of the 98,000 EGMs in New South Wales (Australian Productivity Commission 2010). Gambling operations may be the primary activity of the "club", which is often managed by a private company. As the system has developed over time, a large part of the profit from the machines seems to go to private interests rather than to the "community benefit" which it is supposed to serve (Livingstone 2007).

EGMs have also been provided by charities in Finland, where the Slot Machine Association was, until 2016, formally a conglomerate of associations operating one casino, 20,000 slot machines installed in public places, and (since 2013) an online casino. It contributed approximately one billion EUR for public purposes annually. It was merged with the Finnish State Lottery Company (Veikkaus) in 2017.

The original charitable aim has in many cases been subverted and the funds are used for private-interest purposes (Livingstone 2007), or have turned into important sources of government revenue, as described in Box 10.1.

Gambling enterprises on reserved land owned by tribes of indigenous peoples in North America also illustrate the unanticipated developments, including commercialization, which often follow from carving out special arrangements for "good causes" (see Box 10.2).

Control structures

Regulating ministries and state bodies

Gambling regulation is governed by different administrative levels and branches depending on the jurisdiction in question. A comparative study of European gambling policy models (Polders 1997) found that the body in charge of controlling gambling regulation tends to depend on the arguments

Box 10.1 ONCE for the Blind in Spain

ONCE (Organización Nacional de Ciegos Españoles, i.e., the National Organization of the Blind) was established in 1938 to assist blind people but today provides the Spanish government with revenue, although still contributing some support for the blind. Representatives of ONCE sell lottery tickets across Spain through ONCE kiosks and other vendors. ONCE board members are elected every four years (they are either blind or have impaired vision). In the past ONCE has had a private television channel, a newspaper and a radio station, in addition to hotels and real estate. ONCE also runs projects abroad (e.g., in Haiti). Unemployment has been remarkably low among blind people in Spain, in part due to the activities of ONCE (Giles 2000).

Box 10.2 "Indian casinos": commercial gambling provisions for indigenous reservations in North America

The Indian Gaming Regulatory Act (IGRA), a federal law passed in the United States in 1988, established gambling activities exempt from state tax within Indian reservations, under certain circumstances. Revenues are used to fund tribal government operations and programs, to provide for the general welfare of the Indian tribe and its members, and to promote tribal economic development (Schaap 2010). First Nations communities in Canada have received similar privileges (Williams et al. 2011a).

A total of 237 Indian tribes owned 460 casinos in 2011, generating 26 billion USD in revenue (Fahrenkopf 2012). Indian gambling has led to the resurrection of the Pequot tribe in the state of Connecticut, geographically situated near major population concentrations, after 300 years of extinction (Fromson 2004). The re-invented Pequots now control a gambling business worth over one billion USD per year and operate one of the largest casinos in the United States. Tribes living on reservations far away from big cities are less fortunate (Foderaro 2016). Indian casinos are typically operated under contract by outside gambling enterprises, which view them as lucrative opportunities (Stutz 2014).

that were used in the process of legalizing gambling. If financial concerns or tourism have been predominant, governments prioritize the financial, commercial, and industrial authorities. This has been the case in Germany, Austria, and Portugal. If criminality arguments have been predominant, as in France, governments give priority to criminal justice institutions and ministries of interior affairs.

Many countries have delegated control functions to the administrative branches that allocate public proceeds from gambling for specific purposes. In many countries horse racing is kept separate and placed under the ministries of agriculture, because their returns are directed toward breeding and other forms of support for this rural activity. Often the responsibility is divided between ministries that are expected to minimize gambling-related harm, and others that allocate public revenue from gambling to beneficiaries. Box 10.3 describes the diverse government structures involved in the regulation of gambling in the Nordic countries.

Federal versus state government

Many countries are faced with the question of dividing responsibility for gambling regulation between federal, state, and regional levels of governance,

---

Box 10.3 Nordic structures of gambling regulation

The Norwegian state-owned company, Norsk Tipping, is owned by the Ministry of Culture, and the Ministry of Agriculture and Food owns Norsk Rikstote, a foundation in charge of running tote betting in Norway. The Swedish state-owned company Svenska Spel is controlled by the Ministry of Enterprise and Innovation, and the Horse Racing Totalizator Board has the chair and six members on its Board appointed by the government. In Denmark, the Gaming Authority is established under the Ministry of Taxation. Lotteries in Iceland are operated under licenses given by the Ministry of Justice and Ecclesiastical Affairs (Järvinen-Tassopoulos 2012). The Finnish state-owned gambling monopoly is regulated by the Ministry of Internal Affairs, while gambling funds are redistributed through the Ministry of Education and Culture, Ministry of Health and Social Affairs, and Ministry of Agriculture. The Ministry of Social Affairs and Health has a permanent consulting role on gambling policy from the harm prevention point of view. The Nordic control regimes are under pressure to change, mostly in adaptation to the growing online market.

whereas it is unusual to give local governments authority over these issues. Federal states have taken varying positions regarding the issue. In Australia, the United States, Canada, and Germany, states and provinces have the most authority over gambling. In other countries, such as Mexico, Brazil, and Russia, gambling is considered a federal matter. In Switzerland, national policies regarding gambling are absent, partly because the federal state has a limited role in most policy areas.

Policy examples show that federal management over gambling policies can have some advantages in comparison to state-level governance. The US constitution has conferred strong regulatory powers to states, also extending to online gambling, but the Unlawful Internet Gambling Enforcement Act (passed by the Federal Congress in 2006) could attenuate some stakeholder interests by restricting money transfers related to online gambling (Beem and Mikler 2011). Lack of federal or international regulation may lead to states competing for a comparative advantage by legalizing new games or by reducing tax burdens on providers.

International regulation

Since the 1990s, the internet has turned gambling into an international issue, but the share of responsibilities on an international scale has hardly been discussed. Such responsibilities can be defined within a number of social frames. Money laundering and other illegal activities might point to the United Nations Office on Drugs and Crime as being responsible. Various kinds of sports-related gambling issues could be addressed by sports governance bodies—suggesting perhaps that UNESCO and the International Olympics Committee could become globally responsible. Public health problems (see e.g., Korn and Shaffer 1999) might suggest the jurisdiction of the World Health Organization (Room and Cisneros Örnberg 2014).

So far the international handling of gambling has been managed only by the World Trade Organization (WTO) and the European Union. The former primarily deals with complaints against individual countries for violating international trade law. A WTO decision judged illegal the prohibition by the United States of online gambling offered from offshore (Schneider 2013; Claybrook 2007). So far the United States has ignored the decision. National limits on the supply of gambling services are justified in the WTO context only for the protection of morality, public order, health, and human life, and essential security interests (Trimble 2015).

The EU has gone one step further by adopting a set of principles for online gambling to inform gamblers about the risks, return rates, and their own expenditures; to restrict access to risk groups, and to exclude minors. These principles include ensuring that users have access to help lines and assistance (European Commission 2012). The European Commission has given priority to national control regimes, but they have to be proportionate and cannot discriminate according to national origin or base of the service. States may have to show why a specific regulatory model is better than an alternative in ensuring consumer protection. There are currently no harmonization initiatives (Planzer 2014; Cisneros Örnberg and Tammi 2011).

It is important to note that the organizations regulating international trade became active in this area only after the expansion had occurred. International trade law is therefore not responsible for the increase in and liberalization of national gambling markets.

In the absence of international agreements, many private online operators seek accreditation from independent organizations such as the World Lottery Association or GamCare to demonstrate commitment to social responsibility and also to gain legitimacy (Auer and Griffiths 2013b). In online gambling, systems such as E-Commerce and Online Gaming Regulation and Assurance (eCOGRA) establish minimum standards for consumer protection (including data security issues and responsible gambling), fair gambling (including game rules, certification of equipment, and maintenance of transaction records), and responsible conduct (including anti-money laundering steps and advertising restrictions).

Trimble (2013) has suggested that an International Convention on Online Gambling should be developed under the auspices of the WTO. The agreement would include sections on the exchange of information, enforcement assistance, dispute resolution, cooperation in licensing and standardization, and coordinated "responsible gambling" provisions. However, so far there have been no steps to adopt such an agreement.

The relative benefits of federal regulation in comparison to state-level authority can be extended in support of international regulation. If jurisdictions would be willing to give up some of their control over gambling to cross-jurisdictional or international bodies, this would likely reduce conflicts of interest, diminish competition between states or countries, and increase coherence and information sharing regarding best practices and effective consumer protection.

Whichever form of international regulation should be developed, Gainsbury et al. (2014b) have highlighted the importance of international standards being mandatory rather than voluntary codes of conduct.

Public revenue from gambling

There is considerable variation in how the public revenue from gambling is collected. Methods of collection include taxes, licensing fees, and direct grants to charities and other not-for-profit organizations.

In most cases, gambling taxes are imposed on gross gambling revenue (GGR), which is total wager minus payouts. Besides normal business taxes such as the VAT, there may also be a special tax on admission to gambling venues (especially in the United States), and other fees. In some countries, players' winnings are also taxable. Online gambling presents a particular problem for tax collection. In 2014, the UK introduced a "point-of-consumption" tax of 15%, charged to the game provider when the gambling revenue originates in the UK (HMRC 2013).

Chambers (2011) compared gambling regimes based on how much revenue they produce for governments. States were classified based on their welfare state regime: liberal (United States, Canada, Australia, New Zealand, and the United Kingdom), liberal-corporatist (Ireland, Iceland, Switzerland, Japan, and the Netherlands), corporatist (Spain, Italy, Greece, Germany, Belgium, Luxembourg, Austria, France, and Portugal), and social democratic (Denmark, Finland, Sweden, and Norway). Liberal states allow the most market competition in casinos with a total per capita GGR of 81 USD, social democratic models are the most restrictive with 10 USD and liberal-corporatist and corporatist welfare states are between the two. For EGMs outside casinos the differences are similar, with the exception of Finland and Norway, which had a high EGM availability at the time of the study. As discussed in Chapter 7, Norway has since considerably restricted EGM gambling.

Liberal welfare regimes collect most money from gamblers, but this money may not show in the state budgets or in other contributions to good causes, because private corporations peel off significant profits. In Nevada, for example, gambling companies are only taxed between 3.5% and 6.75% of their profits (Dadayan 2016), and the companies have no obligation to contribute to public funds directly. In the United Kingdom, classified as a liberal welfare state and also a liberal gambling regime, the relative contribution to public funds is low, about 0.6% (Table 10.1). The United Kingdom has wanted to create a system that would attract gambling companies to the country by offering relatively low levels of taxation. Different types of gambling are encouraged in different welfare regimes; state lotteries are important in social democratic welfare states whereas casinos and EGMs are popular in liberal and liberal-corporatist states.

Table 10.1 Importance of public gambling revenue in selected jurisdictions compared to the state budget

Jurisdiction	Public revenue gambling compared to state budget* (percent)	Year	Source
AUSTRALIA (average)	7.8	2015	Australian Gambling Statistics 1989–90 to 2014–15, 32nd edition, 2016
- Victoria	9.6	2015	(percent of state revenue) Australian Gambling Statistics 1989–90 to 2014–15, 32nd edition, 2016
- Western Australia	2.6	2015	(percent of state revenue) Australian Gambling Statistics 1989–90 to 2014–15, 32nd edition, 2016
CANADA (average)	2.2	2013	Responsible Gambling Council 2015
- Alberta	3.5	2013	Responsible Gambling Council 2015
- British Columbia	2.7	2013	Responsible Gambling Council 2015
- Ontario	1.7	2013	Responsible Gambling Council 2015
- Québec	1.2	2013	Responsible Gambling Council 2015
FINLAND	2	2016	Contributions of the gambling monopolies to charities, sports and culture, and gambling taxes compared to state budget.
FRANCE	1.7	2015	Cour des Comptes 2016
GERMANY	1.6	2012	Total public gambling revenues (Fiedler 2016a) compared to federal state budget.
	0.8	2012	Total public gambling revenues compared to federal and state budgets combined (our calculations)
ITALY	2	2012	Gandolfo and De Bonis 2013
MACAU	40	2011	Huang 2011
NORWAY	0.6	2016	Contributions and taxes of Norwegian gambling monopolies compared to state budget.
SWEDEN	1.8	2016	Contributions and taxes of licensed gambling companies and NGOs compared to state budget (Lotteriinspektionen 2015).

Table 10.1 Continued

Jurisdiction	Public revenue gambling compared to state budget* (percent)	Year	Source
UNITED KINGDOM	0.5	2014	Our calculation compared to state budget.
UNITED STATES (average)	2.3	2006	Dadayan et al. 2008
- Nevada	13.4	2006	Dadayan et al. 2008
- West Virginia	8.9	2006	Dadayan et al. 2008
- New Jersey	3.8	2006	Dadayan et al. 2008
- Illinois	4.0	2006	Dadayan et al. 2008
- New York	2.9	2006	Dadayan et al. 2008
- California	0.9	2006	Dadayan et al. 2008

*Sources use various concepts of state budget and/or government revenue. The percentages here refer to the relative size of proceeds from gambling for public purposes, although these may only be partly included in state budgets. The Swedish NGOs with a license do not pay taxes, but their revenue from gambling is included. Averages for the U.S., Australia and Canada are computed on the state/provincial budgets; the federal budget is not in the calculation.

Overall contribution to public funds

The multifarious ways of collecting funds for public use from gambling makes it very difficult to estimate its total volume. Therefore, the following examples must be interpreted as very rough estimations of the relative weight of the industry in the public economy.

Differences between fiscal regimes and in the centralization of government finances limit comparability between countries. For example, the German federal budget is only around 300 billion EUR, whereas the British central government budget is approximately 640 billion EUR. Many sources do not mention which budget they are referring to. For simplicity, we based our calculations on the budgets of the states included in Table 10.1. The figures for public gambling revenues may not be comparable. Sometimes they include "revenue from food, beverage, and other items" in casinos (Responsible Gambling Council 2015), and sometimes not. Direct contributions to charities, sports, etc., are included in the figures for some countries like Finland and Sweden, but only gambling-related taxes are included for others. The UK figure, for example, does not include the direct contributions of society lotteries, but includes the significant revenue from the National Lottery.

Keeping these inconsistencies in mind, the table allows us to conclude that the contributions of gamblers to public finance and good purposes varies a great deal, usually following the per capita amount spent on the activity. The examples of the United States and Australia in particular illustrate that jurisdictions with the widest availability of gambling tend to have high overall public revenue from this source. The United Kingdom is the most notable exception with a figure that we have estimated as 0.6% as compared with its state budget. In many other European countries, public gambling revenues have been of the order of one to two percent as compared with their state budgets.

Australia has the highest total government revenue from gambling among the OECD countries, but variations between its states are significant. Jurisdictions with EGMs in clubs and bars, such as Victoria and the Northern Territory, have the highest overall per-capita tax revenue. Western Australia, with EGMs only in a single casino, has the lowest (Queensland Government Statistician's Office 2016).

Gambling taxes in the United States contribute on average between 2% and 2.5% of revenue for most states (Dadayan 2016), but variation is again great. Nevada has the highest overall tax revenue (over 10%) from gambling, followed by states with a wide variety of different gambling opportunities, including lotteries, "racinos" (race tracks with EGMs), and casinos. North Dakota, Hawaii, Utah, and Oklahoma are the most abstinent states, with zero to 0.1% of revenue from gambling in the state budgets (Walker and Jackson 2011). State revenue largely excludes revenue from Native American gambling operations, although some states have negotiated revenue-sharing agreements with tribes (Dadayan 2016).

Compared to the total amounts of state budgets, several percent may not seem like a high figure, but these are significant amounts in comparison to a number of other sources. For example in Canada, government revenue from gambling exceeded tobacco and alcohol revenue combined by 2003 (Adams et al. 2009), in Australia the average over territories (about 7%) is between returns from tobacco and alcohol. In the United States the gambling revenue corresponds to about one half of the corporate income tax collected by the states (Dadayan et al. 2008). Finland rates highest among European countries, with gambling returns that exceed the returns from tobacco (2.5%) and are slightly smaller than those from alcohol (1.5%). Italy, France, and Norway come close despite the differences in their gambling regimes.

What is the money used for?

Funds collected through gambling create stakeholder interests within the government, and in the sectors that are subsidized. It is likely that dependencies are greater when the subsidies are channeled directly from the game operators instead of the state (Paldam 2008). Particular services and activities may be critically dependent on gambling proceeds. Sports betting has been among the earliest forms of legalized gambling, and consequently government support for sports often comes from this source. Youth work and cultural activities are also often dependent on gambling.

Activities supported by national lotteries seem relatively similar across jurisdictions. For example in Finland, the National Lottery supports sports (28% of proceeds), arts (43%), science (21%), and youth work (10%). The Finnish slot machine association funds NGOs (29%), war veterans (10%), and the state budget (3%). In Norway, sports is the most significant beneficiary (56%), followed by cultural activities (26%), and health and welfare (18%) (Norsk Tipping 2016). In the United Kingdom, figures are quite similar. Health, education, the environment, and charities make up about 40% of funded causes, alongside sports (20%) and cultural heritage (20%). In the United States, the most important beneficiaries of state lotteries are educational institutions, but this source covers less than one percent of their total expenses (Gidluck 2016), and this money may be more than offset by cuts in contributions from state budgets (Summers Robinson et al. 1997).

In many countries support for culture is channeled toward building museums and monuments that then become a cost burden for local communities. A similar issue has been identified in Norway regarding funding for sports. Support has largely been used for the building of sports facilities and venues, but the funds are not sufficient for maintaining them, thus creating a burden on municipalities and sports associations, which in turn seek grants from gambling-related government funds.

Similar problems of inefficiency have arisen when charities are themselves licensed to organize gambling to cover their expenses. A report on Canadian charity lotteries found that only 27% of each dollar raised was retained for funding charity programs. The remainder was used to pay for prizes, marketing, and operational expenses (Thomson and Cheng 2013).

The disadvantages of the dependencies created have been recognized by the Australian Productivity Commission (1999; 2010), suggesting that charitable organizations could collect the funds directly from members and through other activities. Tax exemptions make it difficult to control the use of gambling returns, and it has been estimated that in fact only a minor percentage is used for the designated purposes (Livingstone et al. 2012). Associations and charitable organizations often have close links to political power, which complicates the regulatory functions in view of the public interest (Jensen 2017).

Regime effectiveness in serving the public interest

Different control regimes can and should be evaluated for their ability to protect consumers from gambling harm, to maintain the integrity of games, and to reduce corruption, money laundering, and other gambling-related crime. These are the justifications most commonly used when regulators wish to channel consumption to regulated, national providers.

Protecting consumers from gambling harm

The lowest rates of problem gambling tend to occur in Europe, intermediate rates in North America and Australia, and the highest rates are found in Asia (Williams et al. 2012a). This would suggest that the control regime plays a part. The Court of Justice of the European Union holds the view that monopolies can protect consumers effectively. The Court of Justice of the European Free Trade Association States has similarly held that state-run operations are likely to be better at protecting consumers than business or charity operations (Planzer 2014).

However, there is very little empirical evidence to substantiate these assumptions. One review (Planzer and Wardle 2011) showed no differences between regulatory models in this respect. One comparative study (Planzer et al. 2014) found no significant differences between public monopolies and other regulatory models. However, the sample was small, as only 22 prevalence studies for 12 different European countries were included, and problem gambling prevalence rates are subject to many sources of error that make comparisons unreliable (see Chapter 5).

Other studies have evaluated the impact of regulatory changes in single jurisdictions, but it is not possible to disentangle the impact of changing regimes from the effects of changes in availability that usually accompany the regime change (as was shown in Chapter 7 for Norway, Germany, France, and the UK).

It is likely that any regulatory model can be effective in preventing problem gambling as long as concrete measures are implemented to reduce the amount of gambling and direct gamblers to the least risky types of games and environments.

Integrity of games

The "integrity of games" means assuring consumers that they get what they pay for and know what the price is. Different regulation regimes might be expected to show different results for game integrity, but the interpretation of evidence is difficult. This is because the products provided by gambling operators, including hope and positive subjective experiences, are intangible. As discussed in Chapters 7 and 8, the "price" of the game is usually not known to consumers, and the operators systematically cloak the real chances of winning in their game designs, encouraging false beliefs about controlling chance.

There is little evidence as to which regulatory regimes provide the highest levels of integrity. Only one comparative study has been conducted on the topic (Wiebe and Lipton 2008), concluding that in comparison to prohibition or free market arrangements, licensing regimes with high costs to providers are the most effective way to guarantee that games are fair. The case of France shows similar results. The partial deregulation of online markets in France, from a monopoly system to licensed providers, has helped to increase the transparency of gambling operations, with adequate resources to the national controlling body, ARJEL, to supervise transactions (Cour des Comptes 2016). Other examples show that legalization in itself does not eliminate fraudulent activity. According to one estimate, approximately 250 million AUD (about 190 million USD) was lost between the years 1998 and 2007 through fraudulent actions in Australia (Warfield 2008). For example, match fixing scandals have been uncovered across jurisdictions, irrespective of regulatory models. Finland has been listed as one of the countries with issues in match-fixing and sport-related fraud, along with Poland, the Netherlands, Austria, the Czech Republic, Turkey, and Romania (Spapens 2012), and with Portugal and Italy, countries that do not have a public gambling monopoly (Anderson 2011).

Unregulated gambling, money laundering, and corruption

Preventing unauthorized gambling is one of the major concerns of gambling regulators, both in terms of consumer protection and revenue generation. Studies have found that legalizing gambling will redirect consumers to authorized providers. This may reduce unregulated gambling, but it also attracts new consumers (Spapens 2008b). In some cases, such as in Italy, the rise of legalized gambing was actually accompanied by a parallel rise in different forms of unregulated gambling. The Italian Anti-Mafia Commission (Anti-Mafia Commission 2016) emphasizes that the boundaries between legal and illegal markets are blurred. Illegal organizations penetrate the gambling market by extortion imposed on concessionaires and gambling venues, by the infiltration into the legal market through dummies or shareholding, and by the management of unauthorized betting on websites located in foreign countries.

The line between legal and illegal gambling can be difficult to draw. In the United States, the Unlawful Internet Gambling Act (UIGEA) prohibits online sports betting across state borders, but this has led to the rise of "fantasy sports betting". In these games, people make bets on imaginary teams consisting of real players. Legally the practise is a grey area, but the profits are real. Entry fees paid for this type of betting have been estimated to reach 11 billion USD by 2020 (Matuszewski 2014).

The challenge is to find not only the right regulatory balance, but also to find the means to actively prevent illegal and unregulated gambling opportunities. According to some studies on online gambling, licensing regimes may be the best option to accomplish this (Spapens 2014). License fees provide funding for monitoring and blocking unauthorized competition, and licensed providers can be required to assure consumer safety and integrity of games. By the nature of their set up, government monopolies do not usually have access to such resources (Gainsbury 2012; Marionneau and Järvinen-Tassopoulos 2017).

Money laundering is a major concern for regulatory regimes, being associated with other organized crime. The OECD International Financial Action Task Force has indicated a number of ways in which gambling can be used to disguise the origin of illegally acquired funds. These include inserting money into gambling machines and cashing it out immediately, losing money intentionally to use payouts legally, using third parties to acquire chips, exchanging coins or checks for cash in gambling venues, or using acquaintances within the staff or ownership of the gambling venue. It is possible to launder money in sports, not just by placing bets with criminal proceeds, but also by using illegally gained assets to invest in football clubs, player transfers, advertising contracts, and sponsorship (Financial Action Task Force 2009). The risk of money laundering is diminished in online gambling, as all electronic fund transfers can be recorded. Licensing or monopolization has the potential to reduce the occurrence of money laundering by improving the tracking of monetary transfers due to identification of players (Gainsbury and Wood 2011).

Corruption is another form of malpractice particularly in countries where a substantial part of the business occurs outside legal limits. This attracts corruption of personnel staffing the supervisory institutions, especially the police. In Brazil *Jogo do Bicho* ("the animal game") is an illegal game although a lucrative business for criminals, and the police and politicians have also been implicated because of the large amounts of money involved (Duran 2013).

Jurisdictions with legalized gambling are not free from corruption either, and this seems to apply to all kinds of regimes. In the United States, convictions of state public officials for corruption increased between 1985 and 2000 when casinos were legalized in many US states (Walker and Calcagno 2013). The corrupting influence started a year or two before and continued after legalization. Gambling advocacy groups and operators place large amounts of funding at the disposal of those campaigning for public office in elections (Davis 2006). The power of large gambling-dependent organizations can be considerable, as demonstrated in the successful campaigning against an EGM pre-commitment system by the gambling industry in Australia in 2010–11 (Panichi 2013).

Strictly controlled licensing or a monopoly system, in which gambling regulation is separated from its beneficiaries, may be the best way to prevent corruption. However, without an effective justice system, the choice of regulatory model alone will not solve the issue of corruption or any other gambling-related crime.

Conclusion: the gambling complex

Gambling regulation regimes involve both the public and private sectors, different types of institutions, rules, structures of supervision and ideological principles, and of course involve the investment of money and technology. The gambling complex, as it may be called, impacts on a wide area of social life, far beyond the activity itself and its direct consequences. The extra money that circulates in the gambling complex creates what we called in Chapter 1 the Second Loop: webs of dependencies, vested interests, investments and income that are firmly institutionalized—often based on long traditions, and as a result difficult to change.

Evidence presented in this chapter has shown that strict regulation, whether in monopoly or licensing systems, appears to have the most overall advantages when looking at the comparative efficiency of reducing gambling-related harm and providing revenue to governments, reducing unregulated gambling, assuring the integrity of games, and preventing corruption and crime. Monopoly and strict licensing systems serve these functions well only if they are efficient in their aim at reducing unregulated gambling rather than only offering a legalized alternative. Licensing allows governments to collect resources from licensees to control unauthorized commmerce. Online gambling monopolies exist in the Nordic countries, Luxembourg, Switzerland, and Slovakia, but several of these are moving towards licensing.

With regard to the use of public funds, directing revenue from gambling to general budgets via effective taxation may be a better option than permitting gambling operators to donate pre-tax funds to not-for-profit organizations or public services. This may reduce the conflicts of interest and dependencies of the Second Loop.

Structures of governance, in themselves, do not appear to have much impact on harms; what is important in the structure is the strength and commitment of the agency implementing the regime, and its commitment to the public interest. The location of a responsible state authority within the department structure of the government will also influence the ways in which gambling is considered. Finance ministries expect maximum returns to the state, and possibly contributions to service provision. Administrative structures responsible for commerce, competition, industry, and the labor market, see the gambling industry from the point of view of employment and investments, and see consumer protection as one element in the business environment of the industry. Spending ministries responsible for culture, sports, youth work, public health, social, and leisure services, are keen to maintain and increase their revenues from gambling. Ministries governing the police and criminal justice system seldom address the issues of gambling-related harm to participants in legal gambling (Buhringer et al. 2013). Ministries responsible for public health and social affairs are probably best fitted to focus on gambling-related harm, but even they may eventually derive funding for services, treatment, education, and research from gambling proceeds (Adams 2016). Gambling licensing and regulatory enforcement units thus need to be institutionally insulated from such interests.

However regulation is organized, it needs to be backed up by an autonomous and transparent regulatory and court system, and by a body that is not dependent on gambling revenues, either public, non-governmental or private. In this way the broader considerations of justice and distributional effects, included in our concept of the public interest, that go beyond direct harm caused by gambling, and beyond specific risk factors related to games and gambling environments, can be objectively assessed and accounted for. These considerations should be clearly stated in the mandate of the supervisory authority.

Independent community-based advocacy, including church groups, community alliances, and political parties, can be an important force challenging government complicity with gambling, and may offer new possibilities to reduce vested interests in gambling (Adams et al. 2009). Alliances of such interested non-governmental organizations at local, national, and international levels can also be positive forces acting in the public interest.

Policy makers should place less emphasis on the balance between the benefits and the harm from gambling and instead ask whether the public services thereby funded could be resourced in other, less problematic and less harmful ways.

Chapter 11

Treatment and early intervention services

People with gambling problems in many countries can now receive help from a variety of mental health and social services, which have been specifically developed for them. These services need to be considered at both the individual and population levels if a comprehensive public interest approach is to be applied to gambling problems. This chapter reviews research on the treatment of gambling disorders and gambling problems, not only in terms of their positive effects on individual gamblers and their families, but also in the context of larger systems and their population-level impact.

A key purpose of treatment is to help people change their gambling behavior and address their gambling-related problems. This chapter focuses on services that have been evaluated scientifically, and the ways in which they produce benefit for the individual as well as society. The goals of such services are diverse and may include initiating abstinence from gambling, maintaining abstinence once achieved, reducing the amount or frequency of gambling, and addressing problems with family relations, mental health, personal finances, criminal justice, and employment. Services vary considerably within and across societies, but they all share the assumption that individual-level behavior change (e.g., in coping responses, relapse prevention skills) will translate into lower rates of gambling, gambling problems, unemployment, and criminal activity. In addition to self-help organizations and financial counselling, treatment for problem and pathological gambling is delivered in both non-residential and residential settings.

Treatment outcome research

Professional treatment for individual gambling problems is a relatively recent innovation. Meta-analyses of outcome evaluation studies published in the second half of the 1990s (Blaszczynski and Silove 1995; López-Viets and Miller 1997; National Research Council 1999) all concluded that this field was at a very early stage of development. They did, however, draw the encouraging conclusion, not always accepted previously, that positive change was possible for people who entered treatment for gambling problems. One of the best early studies, conducted in Minnesota, United States with 274 gamblers using a multi-modal treatment approach (Stinchfield and Winters 1996), reported abstinence rates of 43% at six months' follow-up and 42% at 12 months, with an additional 20 and 24% gambling in a controlled way. Later reviews, such as that of Toneatto and Ladouceur (2003), reached the same positive conclusion, that gambling disorder is a treatable condition.

Since then, the treatment research literature has been expanding rapidly but still gives every impression of being at a very early stage of development. Two more recent reviews are illustrative.

The first is a Cochrane-style review of psychological therapies by Cowlishaw et al. (2012). Cochrane reviews explore the evidence for and against the effectiveness and appropriateness of medical treatments as well as social and psychological interventions. The review included randomized trials, where clients assigned to therapy were compared to untreated controls or referral to Gamblers Anonymous (GA). The 14 trials included 11 studies of cognitive behavior therapy (CBT), four studies of motivational interviewing (MI) therapies, and two studies of integrative therapies. CBT is a type of psychological therapy which is used to help people recognize and change thoughts, feelings, and behaviors that are causing gambling problems, and to learn alternative responses to tempting and difficult situations. In particular, CBT therapists help clients abandon cognitive illusions about winning at gambling. MI refers to a counseling approach that attempts to enhance intrinsic motivation to change gambling behavior by helping clients to explore and resolve their ambivalence about gambling.

Data from nine studies indicated benefits of CBT in the period immediately following treatment, but the review concluded that little is known about whether the effects of CBT are lasting. Preliminary evidence for some benefits from MI therapy was found in terms of reduced gambling behavior, although not necessarily other symptoms of problem gambling. In general, few studies provided data on secondary symptoms of depression and anxiety, or other outcomes such as gambling cognitions. The trials varied in quality. For example, some provided limited or no description of the method of random allocation, which may have deviated from an ideal protocol. Several studies managed attrition through 'completers only' analysis, which may also overestimate the effects of treatment. There was further variability in the use of allocation concealment and blinding of outcome assessors. The authors of the review commented that much of the evidence comes from studies with multiple limitations, so the available data may reflect overestimates of treatment efficacy. Although more comprehensive and rigorous than earlier reviews (e.g., Toneatto and Ladouceur

2003), the Cowlishaw et al. (2012) review produced findings that were generally consistent with prior reviews, which had argued for the efficacy of psychological therapy for the treatment of problem gambling, specifically CBT.

The second review (Petry 2005) again reported that CBTs were the ones most widely researched, with studies from the United States, Australia, and Sweden. Overall, these studies reached positive conclusions but they were not without methodological limitations. Most relied on "waitlist control groups," which consist of participants who are put on a waiting list to receive the intervention after the active treatment group does. Waitlist control groups provide an ethical alternative to withholding treatment entirely, but they may create expectations that there is no need to make a change until the active treatment begins, and thereby inflate the difference between the intervention and control groups. In addition, they make it impossible to assess comparatively long-term outcomes because of the ethical imperative to provide needed treatment.

In one study a CBT workbook combined with MI resulted in significant reductions in gambling, in comparison to a waitlist control group (Hodgins et al. 2001). Another study by the same group found that the workbook-only participants were less likely to reduce losses and pathological gambling symptoms in the 24-month follow-up period (Hodgins et al. 2004). Results support the value of brief treatments but also indicate that more treatment may confer even greater benefits.

Other studies have evaluated brief advice with motivational treatments alone. For example, one was conducted with college students with gambling problems and another with patients who screened positive at medical clinics and alcohol and drug treatment programs (Petry et al. 2008). In those studies, the brief advice, consistent with harm minimization principles, included the following caveats: 1) gamble for fun, not to make money; 2) gamble only what you can afford to lose; 3) set a dollar limit each time you gamble; 4) set a time limit each time you gamble; 5) leave checks, credit cards, and ATM cards at home; 6) take your winnings home; and 7) remember the odds are always in favor of the house. Results showed that single session interventions can be effective, suggesting that more extensive treatments (e.g., combining MI and CBT) do not improve outcomes beyond single session interventions in non-treatment-seeking populations. A series of Canadian studies also showed benefits of single session motivational interventions (Cunningham et al. 2009; 2012).

Petry (2005) concluded that psychosocial treatments are efficacious in reducing gambling problems in the short term, but the specific types of treatment that are most efficacious remain to be determined. Because many problem and pathological gamblers recover without formal interventions, and many others substantially decrease gambling once they decide to initiate treatment, the long-term efficacy of even the most promising interventions remains to be demonstrated. Another concern is the lack of an agreed standard for determining outcomes, which have included self-reports of urges to gamble, actual days gambling, amounts wagered, and symptoms of pathological gambling. Furthermore, therapist differences in training, adherence, and competence have been assessed in only a few studies.

Although the systematic reviews have largely been confined to studies of psychological therapies for individuals, those are not the only methods that have been used to help people with gambling problems. Petry (2005) also refers to GA, which originated in California in the late 1950s, growing to over 500 chapters in the United States by the late 1980s (Lesieur 1990) and now operating in 51 countries. Although based on the principles of Alcoholics Anonymous (AA), and other 12-Step mutual-help organizations (Humphreys et al. 2004), Browne (1991) concluded from a large observational study that GA placed far greater emphasis than AA upon members' financial circumstances, on the need to make a personal financial inventory, and on the centrality of excessive gambling as the problem (rather than character and spirituality). Treatment evaluation reviews have been cautious about GA. One early study in Scotland (Stewart and Brown 1988) suggested that dropout rates were high and abstinence rates low. One non-randomized study (Petry 2003) did find a higher abstinence rate for those attending both GA and professional treatment compared to those who attended professional treatment alone, but otherwise studies of the effectiveness of GA have been absent. It is therefore difficult to draw conclusions (Schuler et al. 2016). Nevertheless, if the AA research can serve as the model, several large-scale randomized studies have shown that 12-Step programs like AA are as effective or even more effective than professional treatment (Walsh et al. 1991; Babor and Del Boca 2003). The same considerations may apply to GA as to AA, where "... scientific skepticism ... has given way ... to a more humble acceptance of the limitations of professional treatment and a greater awareness of the positive role that mutual-help can play for large numbers of people" (Orford et al. 2003b, 227).

Medications have also been used in the treatment of gambling problems. A recent review by Bullock and Potenza (2015) notes that medications investigated for their efficacy and tolerability in the treatment of problem gambling have included opioid antagonists, mood stabilizers, serotonin reuptake inhibitors, and glutamatergic drugs. Medications considered to be effective in the treatment of substance use disorders and other psychiatric conditions that can co-occur with problem gambling have also been investigated. Although most trials to date have only examined short-term outcomes, the most robust data exist for opioid antagonists such as naltrexone and nalmefene. The data also suggest that SSRIs (selective serotonin reuptake inhibitors) and mood stabilizers, particularly lithium, may be helpful in certain groups of people with gambling problems. They further suggest that combinations of pharmacotherapy and psychological therapy warrant additional investigation.

Services for family members

Estimates of the average number of other people affected for every one person with a gambling disorder vary widely. The Australian Productivity Committee (1999) suggested a figure of seven others, while the 2010 British Gambling Prevalence Survey (Wardle et al. 2011b) suggested four family relatives. Even a conservative estimate of two people so affected—mostly wives, female partners, mothers, and fathers—would suggest that affected family members need services at least as much as people with gambling disorder themselves (Velleman et al. 2015). Services involving family members can be grouped into three categories (Orford et al. 2005): 1) working with gamblers and family members together; 2) interventions that help family members to encourage their problem gambling relatives to enter treatment or to continue to engage in treatment; and 3) helping family members in their own right.

A recent non-randomized Spanish study involving 675 men with gambling disorder found greater engagement in and reduced drop-out from treatment among those for whom a concerned significant other was involved in their treatment (Jiménez-Murcia et al. 2016). A number of uncontrolled, small sample, and case studies have also suggested promising results from treatments involving family members in terms of outcomes for family members themselves. In one study of a coping skills training program, the treatment group showed significantly greater improvement in coping skills and reductions in depression and anxiety than a wait-list control group (Rychtarik and McGillicuddy 2006). Another study compared a minimal intervention, in which family members received a self-help workbook based on behavioral principles, with a no-treatment control group (Hodgins et al. 2007). Both groups showed significant improvements in psychological distress, consequences of gambling, relationship satisfaction, and engagement of the gambler in treatment, but those assigned to the minimal treatment were significantly more satisfied with the program. Another approach, intended for affected family members in their own right, and producing promising results (George and Bowden-Jones 2015), is the 5-Step Method (Copello et al. 2010; Orford 2017).

Accessibility and adequacy of treatment services

Despite promising findings, treatment for problem gambling research lags far behind the research conducted on alcohol and drug treatment. Improving the methodology of controlled trials and increasing the volume of such studies may be one way forward. But attention might also be paid to broader issues concerning the availability of treatment. Lessons learned from the alcohol and drug fields suggest that the wrong research questions have been asked (Orford 2008). Gambling treatment evaluation research tends to take a familiar and conventional form, testing the efficacy of a named treatment for individual people with gambling problems by comparing it with a control condition. But simply asking whether one named treatment, such as CBT, is as good or better than another, may divert attention from more relevant questions about access to help and questions to do with crucial change processes common to a range of treatment types (Gifford et al. 2006). Since conventional gambling treatment research seems to be at a relatively early stage, there is an opportunity to start by asking the right questions rather than wrong ones. Specifically, issues that need to be investigated include: 1) how to provide sufficient and accessible help for people affected by gambling; 2) how to make sure that help is adequate and acceptable; 3) which therapeutic processes account for the behavior change; and 4) where best to provide help.

Availability and accessibility of help. Currently treatment provision is sparse and inadequate, even in well-resourced countries (Meyer et al. 2009). In less resourced countries, the situation is likely to be even worse. This global lack of treatment provision should be set against what is known so far about the prevalence of gambling disorder (see Chapter 5). In Britain, for example, surveys (e.g., Wardle et al. 2011a) have suggested that gambling problem prevalence is of the same order as the prevalence of problems related to the misuse of illicit drugs. The latter, unlike gambling disorder, is recognized as a major public health problem for which health authorities have a responsibility to provide treatment.

Adequacy and acceptability. Even if treatment were more widely available, the majority of people with gambling disorder may be reluctant to engage with it. A number of studies have found that the secrecy and stigma associated with having a gambling problem account for the small proportion of those seeking help among those who could benefit from treatment (Hing et al. 2016; Horch and Hodgins 2015). In the Czech Republic, for example, it has been estimated that less than 5% of pathological gamblers were receiving treatment in 2012 (Szczyrba et al. 2015). Early and preventive interventions targeted at risky gambling may therefore be as important as treatments clearly designated for problem gambling (Petry et al. 2008).

Therapeutic processes. An effective treatment system is likely to embrace a variety of approaches, not all of which would necessarily be recognized as "treatment", ranging from hospital or community residential facilities at the more intensive end of the spectrum, to brief, early interventions, telephone helplines, and online support at the other extreme. Gambling helplines and e-help for gambling have been established in the Nordic countries, the Netherlands, Britain, Australia, and the United States (Griffiths et al. 1999; Goudriaan 2014; Rodda et al. 2014; National Research Council 1999; Rossow and Hansen 2016; Tammi et al. 2015). A recent Australian controlled trial found an internet-based CBT program to be more efficacious than either a wait-list control or an active comparison condition comprising monitoring, feedback, and control (Casey et al. 2017). Ideally there should be a variety of ways in which people can obtain appropriate help, advice or an opportunity to discuss their concerns about their own gambling, or about someone else's gambling.

Where treatment should be located. One suggestion is that treatment should be located within substance misuse services, since there is much in common between problem gambling and substance problems. This is currently the model for gambling treatment delivery in a number of countries including France, the Netherlands, Finland, Norway, and Brazil (Goudriaan 2014; Rossow and Hansen 2016; Tammi et al. 2015; Tavares 2014; Valleur 2015). Another possibility is that general medical and social services should be the main providers. As shown in Chapters 3 and 6, for many people gambling problems are associated with mental disorders, physical health problems, domestic abuse, family problems, and poverty. Therefore, treatment for gambling problems must be well integrated with services that deal with those health and social problems. One obvious approach that is prominent in the Nordic countries is to locate gambling services in the social welfare system that is typically managed by trained social workers. A third possibility is to provide financial counseling for persons with debt problems related to gambling. A fourth solution is to include gambling issues in the law enforcement, crime prevention, and legal counseling systems, as these problems often involve crime or are criminogenic. Finally, help may be incorporated into services for children and young persons, as the prevalence of gambling problems is known to be as high if not higher among adolescents than among adults (Orford et al. 2013).

Each of these choices involves a similar limitation. They address the problems of their clients from the particular perspective of the system in which they belong: addictions, health, welfare, debt, crime, or child and adolescent issues. As problem gambling is a behavioral complex with many dimensions, a helping service should be focused on gambling and cover several or perhaps all of these perspectives. In addition, service providers who are specialized in other areas should be trained and encouraged to recognize an underlying gambling problem and to refer their clients to adequate forms of help.

Research needs to address the question of whether help for gambling problems is equally available for adolescents as for adults, for women as for men (discussed by Kaufman et al. 2016), for affected family members as well as for gamblers, and for minority groups as well as for members of majority groups. As the reach of transnational gambling companies extends to low- and middle-income countries, the extent of accessible treatment will require policy, as well as research, attention.

System level issues

Beyond questions relating to the nature of treatment and their evaluated outcome effects, it is critical to address further system level issues such as the affordability of services as well as how they are organized, funded, and managed.

For example, in Brazil a small number of specialized gambling treatment services are available at the Federal University and the Institute of Psychiatry in São Paulo, plus two others, all in the south and south-east of the country, leaving the poorer areas of the country without specialist services (Tavares 2014). In many other countries, services are available only to a limited part of the population, often beyond the reach of population segments in which they are most needed.

Funding for services can be allocated by governments, by non-governmental organizations or by the private sector. Funding arrangements reflect societal values, historical traditions, and the division of power in the governance structures. Funding priorities and decisions have an impact on accessibility, types of interventions offered, and probably also outcomes. In countries with a private health insurance industry (e.g., Switzerland, Germany, and the United States), funding policy also affects interventions covered by insurance, which will reflect in part public policy choices made by government regulators. Most countries use tax revenues, user fees, and private insurance to pay for gambling treatment services. Tax funding is more important in high income countries, whereas out of pocket financing is more common in poorer countries. Many countries use a part of the extra returns from gambling activities, the rent, for funding problem gambling services. In Britain, for example, the government has handed responsibility for treatment and research to the gambling industry, which raises a small amount of money annually for those purposes, via a voluntary levy on the industry (Orford 2012). Nearly all gambling treatment services, including one specialized clinic within the National Health Service, are funded in this way. A national non-governmental organization that provides face-to-face and phone-line counselling services is financed by the gambling industry with the attendant conflicts of interest and moral jeopardy which that entails (Adams 2008; Livingstone and Adams 2016).

Decisions regarding treatment services are constrained by two important factors. The first concerns priorities in other systems of public service provision, and the division of labor between them. An example is laws specifying what happens to persons with gambling problems, be it punishment, behavioral rehabilitation, denial of access to gambling, health services, addiction treatment, or some combination of these. The other factor is the characteristics of the gambling population. It includes the economic resources of gamblers, the types of gambling problems they are experiencing, and their risk awareness. These factors depend not only on treatment services but on policies that regulate the provision of gambling opportunities.

The need for and provision of treatment services are therefore part of the bigger picture of the system in which treatment is embedded. The tangible aspects of the treatment system alone do not determine their efficiency and effectiveness. These aspects include the number and type of facilities (e.g., clinics, hotlines, internet help sites), the programs delivered in those facilities (e.g., diagnostic assessment, risk reduction and financial counselling, psychotherapy), and the characteristics of personnel in those programs (e.g., certified counselors, social workers, psychiatrists, recovering peer helpers). Less tangible system qualities may be as important as the structural resources of a system. To the extent that services are adapted to the forms of gambling that are offered and most used, and are accessible, coordinated, affordable, voluntary, and not stigmatizing, they are likely to be more effective (Babor et al. 2008).

Structural resources and system qualities, along with the characteristics of the gambling population, combine to produce two important outcomes. The first and most obvious outcome, covered earlier, is the impact on the service recipients themselves (both gamblers and affected others such as close family members). The second is the impact on the population as a whole, including those who do not have a gambling problem. Population impact can be expected in many domains, including public health (e.g., incidence of depression and suicide), criminal justice (e.g., amount of embezzlement and cyber-crime), social welfare (e.g., domestic violence) and finances (e.g., unemployment and disability costs).

Conclusion

We began this chapter by summarizing what is known about the outcome effectiveness of specific treatments for problem gambling, drawing particularly on the findings of two systematic reviews. The provisional conclusions are the following: gambling disorder is treatable; cognitive behavior therapy has been most studied and has been the most supported; and single session and other brief treatments may be as effective as more intensive interventions. Little evidence is available on the effectiveness of treatment or other assistance for family members and others adversely affected by someone's gambling. The field is at an early stage and lacks the research that would be necessary to gauge how much more effective treatment is compared to no treatment, or whether one treatment is superior to another.

Treatment research which concentrates narrowly on the relative effectiveness of named treatments needs to be complemented with studies of the wider context in which treatment is offered. The role played by the mutual-help organization Gamblers Anonymous, the importance of help for family members affected by their relatives' excessive gambling, and the existence of medications that have been used in the treatment of gambling disorder, need to be investigated more systematically.

A major conclusion from research in this area is that in many parts of the world treatment for gambling problems is sparse or non-existent, and even in better resourced countries treatment availability is patchy and engagement in treatment is low, probably in part due to the secrecy and stigma associated with gambling problems. This situation raises questions about the need for service planning when gambling opportunities are increased, including the funding of these services, and about the ability of treatment services to even minimally address the problems linked to gambling.

Treatment services need to be considered in the context of larger systems, and their ability to have a population-level impact in the absence of other policy measures needs to be questioned. To date, population-wide impacts of treatment have not been demonstrated in the critical areas of need, such as public health, criminal justice, social welfare, and finances. Gambling treatment services should never be expected to eliminate a nation's gambling problem, but if properly organized and funded they could make a contribution to the reduction of gambling-related mental disorder, crime, and damage to family life.

Chapter 12

Summary and conclusions: gambling policy and the public interest

The public interest approach to gambling

The public interest approach to gambling sets its main goal the same way as generally accepted public health policy—it is to promote the health and well-being of the general population. It does not rest on judgments of the moral worth of the activity, or of the belief systems that it might be seen to violate—religious, moral or otherwise. The public interest approach aims to make plain the ways in which gambling contributes to human suffering, even misery, without taking a stand on the wealth and happiness that it may bring to some. Throughout human history, and until quite recently, gambling has been subject to criticism, even bans, on many theological and moral grounds that have largely lost their salience in those parts of the world where the activity has developed into a mass entertainment industry. As an activity and an industry, gambling is still seen critically by the majority of the population in countries where opinion surveys have been conducted, but the public interest argument here accounts for this fact only on the side, not in the role of being its advocate.

The evidence from the chapters of this book leads us to conclude that public interest oriented gambling policy must recognize three basic facts. First, gambling has redistributing effects, some benign and some malign, but these two cannot easily be separated from each other. The benign effects are those that help fund necessary social activities—community life, assistance of the needy, health care, youth work, and many others. The malign effects are those that make the poor even poorer and the unhappy even unhappier. The policy question here should be whether the benign effects could be attained in some other way. Second, gambling is even more concentrated in a very small group of heavy users than most other harmful or risky consumer practices. A very large proportion of these people are those who can least afford to fund the benign effects, being themselves in need of help and support. Third, it is an activity that contributes to producing harm and suffering even when it cannot be identified as causing them. Gambling problems co-occur with many other vulnerabilities, and policy considerations should recognize this fact independently of the causal role of gambling in them. *Redistribution of wealth, concentration of the cost on a very small fragment of the population, and reinforcement of other vulnerabilities make gambling policy an issue of distributive justice.*

Gambling expansion, government regulation and the Second Loop

Gambling has been viewed as immoral in many religious and ethical systems, and still is so in many parts of the world. Its expansion from limited elite pastimes and local charity raffles, first to restricted national lotteries and betting games, and then to a commercial activity on a mass scale, is a unique and recent historical development. It started in the 1980s, at the time when global financial markets were deregulated, accelerated after the turn of the century, and covers mainly North America, Europe, and the Asia Pacific region, so far leaving behind most of South America and Africa, and also Russia and mainland China. It is dominated by globally operating multinational companies based in the United States, the United Kingdom, Austria, Hong Kong, Australia, and Macao, often through countries with low taxation and relaxed regulation, including Antigua, Gibraltar, and Malta.

The expansion is coupled with radical changes in governments' approach to regulation. They have felt the need to bring gambling under government control to avoid tax evasion and competition from abroad, and to assure consumer protection, including trust and transparency as well as adherence to responsible gambling codes. The availability of gambling on the internet is often felt to put pressure on governments to liberalize their regulatory systems, but it must be noted that the gambling expansion began before online gaming became a relevant part of the market. Internet gambling still covers only a minor share of the total gambling volume in most countries, whereas a substantial part of land-based gambling takes place outside of the regulated market, for example in India.

It is not possible to determine if liberalized regulation is the cause of the gambling expansion or a reaction to it. In most cases it is probably both. To the extent that free trade agreements under the World Trade Organization and the European Union have included gambling on their agenda, it has occurred only after the expansion.

Many governments have justified the expansion of gambling availability by dedicating some of the "rent" or tax from the increased gambling to "good causes". This justification has had a double function for them:

- it provides an ethical cover for legitimizing an activity which many citizens remain queasy about;
- it raises money for government-supported activities in circumstances where they are reluctant to cover the activities' cost with taxes.

As a consequence, the good causes supported become a constituency in need of continued revenue from the activity. These dependencies constitute what we called in Chapter 1 the Second Loop in gambling policy. Increased gambling creates groups whose income and activities are funded from this source, and any regulations that may cut back gambling volume will arouse concerns about maintaining the status quo.

The two vicious cycles of gambling policy

Gambling is practiced by large proportions of the population in all countries where it is commercially available. The distribution of those participating in the activity, on the scale of time or money spent, is skewed, so that a very small proportion of the gamblers are in the high end, the majority in the middle, and then there is a varying proportion of those who do it very little if at all. The distribution among those who gamble at all is continuous, so that heavy users do not constitute a separate group of addicts or pathological individuals. Those at the high end of the scale contribute the largest share of the total money spent. In most studies the group of heavy users spending close to one half of the total is a smaller fraction of the population than for other behaviors, for example alcohol consumption. Problematic consequences experienced also primarily fall on a very small group of very heavy gamblers, often of the order of one to two percent. These consequences are costly to society, and should be seen as a deduction from the society's revenues from the activity. This is what we call the First Loop or vicious cycle of gambling policy.

The epidemiological studies we have reviewed show that the small minority of problem gamblers do not represent the population segments that can best bear the cost burden of the First Loop, nor the funding interests that constitute the Second Loop. At least one half of the individuals who contribute the largest share of revenues for charitable purposes through gambling are themselves poor, with low educational background, mentally ill, addicted or otherwise problem substance users, physically sick, or have several of these vulnerabilities. This is the case across many different types of populations, gambling environments, and types of games, with the exception that internet gamblers tend to have a higher educational background than land-based gamblers. People with high incomes spend more on gambling than low-income groups, but the latter, on average, spend a larger share of their means on gambling. Gambling-based charity is therefore a larger burden on the needy than on those who have more wealth to share with them, and a particularly large burden on a low-income subgroup of heavy gamblers.

The most efficient forms of gambling for revenue collectors are EGMs and periodic lotteries, the most and least addictive types of games. EGMs cause most of the harm that is related to heavy gambling, lotteries the least. On the other hand, lotteries—especially state lotteries—have the lowest return rates and are played by the poorest people, and they are thus a particularly regressive way of taxing income earners.

Problematic gambling adversely affects not only the gambler, but also a number of people around him or her—estimates range from an average of five to 17 people. The burden is financial, but understandably cuts deep also into interpersonal relationships, trust, emotional stress, and issues of health and welfare generally. Children are affected in many ways, one being an elevated risk of becoming themselves problem or even pathological gamblers.

Problem and pathological gamblers are a very small proportion of the total population, and even of those who participate in gambling at all, at any one time. Research has shown, however, that turnover of individuals within this small population is very high. Economic and personal disasters eliminate some of the heaviest players from the market, but new individuals take their place. This is one of the issues in the epidemiology of gambling problems that needs more research attention, but it is obvious that a high turnover implies a much larger life-time experience of gambling problems than cross-sectional prevalence figures in population surveys suggest.

Given these well-established downsides, politicians and policy-makers should carefully consider to what extent gambling is the only or the preferred way of supporting public services and good causes. Instead of asking whether and to what extent gambling can be seen as a cause of the problems that heavy users suffer from, they must question to what extent should societies lay the cost of their welfare on the most vulnerable and weak. Instead of asking what are the costs and benefits to the whole society, policymakers should pay close attention to who gets the benefits and which population segments bear most of the cost while being themselves also most in need of support.

A further consideration should be given to the powerful vested interests that are created by the support for good causes. The uses for which public revenues from gambling are allocated do not mainly serve the needs of the heavy-using minority. In many cases the contributions only cover a small proportion of the activities covered, as in culture, social services, and education. Still, some providers of these activities may be heavily dependent on this particular funding source. The political process involved in choosing the causes tends to ensure that the causes will have considerable policy influence in arguing against restrictions that would reduce the flow of revenue to support them.

Gambling as business

In this book we have brought up many economic indicators of the volume of the gambling business. The numbers are impressive, and lead many to believe that gambling can be economically stimulating—an especially important outcome in regions that are industrially underdeveloped or otherwise weak in economic resources. The evidence should provoke caution whenever this justification of support for the activity is considered. Gambling is what Adams (2016) calls an extractive industry. It needs a technical infrastructure, it involves services and exchangeable commodities other than the games, but the far greatest part of the industry in monetary terms is the transfer of money from losing gamblers to winning gamblers and from all gamblers to the operators, the state, and the beneficiaries from the surplus. The pleasures of the experience are there, but they are transitory, while the damage persists. It has been observed in many studies that casino destinations tend to push away rather than attract other economic activities.

Gambling, fraud, and crime

Protecting consumers against fraud, eliminating gambling-related crime, fighting tax evasion, and providing safe gambling environments are important considerations in designing legalized gambling regimes. They are also in the interest of the legal industry itself.

The many examples presented in this book show, however, that legalizing national markets does not in itself provide a shield against abuses. Growing legal markets do not necessarily extinguish illegal competition; on the contrary, they may spill over to demand for unregulated services. Regulated licensees tend to develop their own interests in growth and new business opportunities, including participation in global competition, rather than simply substituting their own services for unregulated markets. Depending on the political culture and their position in departmental structures, government monopoly agencies can also develop and pursue such interests.

There is no guarantee that an institutionalized gambling market by itself eliminates fraud, corruption or crime. Policymakers and politicians should therefore attempt to see fraud and crime prevention as a separate and independent issue that cannot be answered simply by more liberal approaches to legal gambling.

Prevention of gambling problems

Those defending national policies against unregulated markets and foreign competition often justify restrictive regulation by appealing to its preventive functions. This argument has some validity: globally operating corporations have little interest in and responsibility for harm prevention if it does not improve their own economic performance. The effectiveness of national regulations in harm prevention depends on their aims and their implementation to achieve these ends.

This book has reviewed the evidence on how regulations on availability do and do not influence the activity itself, and its harmful effects. Caution has been necessary in drawing conclusions. As a general rule, the consumption distribution is skewed, as could be expected from other behaviors. This implies that the average volume of gambling in a population is positively related to heavy use; the prevalence of problem gambling and harm moves up and down together with how much gambling takes place in a population. Regulating the availability is therefore an important instrument for public interest-oriented policy, but three other factors behind simple correlations must also be taken into consideration. The intensity and harm potential of different games is relevant; different subpopulations have different risk potentials and varying capacities to face them; and both of these factors have effects on the distribution of the economic benefits from the activity as well as on who will bear the cost and suffering from it.

We have also identified methods of regulating game features, environments, and contexts in a way that will minimize harm, as well as techniques that the industry uses to maximize its turnover and profits. The research on how game characteristics, casino designs, and other techniques attract money from gamblers is mostly not publicly available. The evidence we have reviewed supports some generalizations concerning what works to reduce the damage. As a general rule, measures that regulate the features of the games and the environments of play are more powerful and more accepted than those that are aimed at the gamblers. Efficient harm minimization techniques are those that set limits to game intensity, inducements, access to games, and access to cash while gambling, whereas information, persuasion, self-assessment, and other personality-based responsible gambling tools mainly serve the interests of game providers. Efficient pre-commitment and limit setting tools are those that are universally applied, mandatory, based on behavior, and implemented with personalized registration across the accessible gambling offered.

The main obstacle to the potential success of such efforts lies in the epidemiological facts presented in this book. Preventing gambling-related harm is not possible without limiting the overall volume of the activity, because in gambling, even more than in other risk-prone behaviors, the problem users are those who bring in the largest share of the money to the trade. Few gambling-related problems are caused by casual recreational gamblers, but only a very few of those who actually are heavy gamblers get away without harm to themselves, to their family, and to their community and society.

Optimum choices in regulating the gambling market

National gambling markets can be organized in several different ways. The market can be run as a government monopoly, usually responsible to a government department or ministry. It can be run by private interests under license and regulated by government authorities. Or the government can license and regulate charitable or other non-profit organizations to be the market actors.

Each of these arrangements has its advantages and drawbacks. From the point of view of the public interest, it is more important as to how well the arrangements separate the regulation of the market from economic interests, both public and private, than which of these structures is actually chosen. It is almost certainly a mistake to lodge the monopoly or licensing agency in the same branch of government that uses the gambling revenue or distributes it to beneficiaries. Such an arrangement increases the likelihood that maximizing revenue from gambling will take priority over minimizing social harm. Likewise, if the market is to be run by a government monopoly, it is wise to have it supervised by a distinct regulating body separated from the monopoly. Legal provisions should give the regulatory agency the power over how many licenses of different varieties are issued, over where retail shops and other outlets are located (including web outlets), and over the conditions of sale in them. The independent control agency should also have control over the extent and content of advertising and promotion of gambling products.

The need for an international public interest agreement on gambling control

With the growth of the globalized gambling industry, national markets are increasingly entering the agendas of international trade agreements, which have the power to set limits on national regulatory policies. For the moment it is not possible to expect any international arrangements either to limit the growth of the industry or the harm it inflicts on populations. The regulative functions and responsibilities to this effect will no doubt remain in the hands of nation states, federal or unitary. Even the European Union free trade policy accepts national governments' functions to prevent harm abuse, and crime, as well as to protect the consumer. However, it does not allow the use of gambling as an extra source of public revenue.

An international agreement needs to be negotiated that includes provisions guaranteeing signatory countries the ability to control their domestic markets in the public interest, even if this could be interpreted as a barrier or limit on trade. Responsibility for implementation of such an agreement could be invested in international organizations such as the World Health Organization, the United Nations Office on Drugs and Crime (UNODC) or the United Nations Educational, Scientific and Cultural Organization (UNESCO).

Conclusion and recommendations

Global gambling expansion is a unique and recent historical development. From local and national charitable action, gambling has developed into a mainstream leisure activity that generates considerable profits for the producer industries, tax revenues for governments, and income for charitable and civil organizations. It is coupled with government policies, mostly at the national, state, and federal level. Decisions on regulations are often seen as necessary adaptations to gambling promotions from abroad or from the unregulated market, but they always have a bearing on how the field develops, what its consequences are and how the benefits and costs are distributed in society. When such decisions are made, the following points should be taken into consideration:

◆ The escalation of the industry generates its own momentum and is difficult to reverse. Every step towards further expansion requires immediate attention from public authorities, policymakers, and the international research community.

◆ Problem gambling has elements of addiction and a psychiatric disorder, but these are not the causes of its consequences. Even pathological gambling, the most serious degree of the problem, should not be primarily handled within the medical model. Social and environmental considerations are critical in the prevention and remediation of gambling problems in society.

◆ Gambling transfers money from players to operators, governments, and "good cause" beneficiaries. Policy should always take into consideration the distribution of costs and benefits between different groups of players and other actors.

◆ A very small part of the population and of those who gamble account for a very large share of the total spending. Preventive policy that aims at reducing their risk of harm will have to accept that that policy will most likely also reduce the total volume of the trade.

◆ Problem gambling co-occurs frequently with mental and physical health problems, substance use, smoking, poverty, family problems, suicide risk, and criminal records. The direction of causality between gambling and these co-morbidities cannot always be determined with certainty, but they should be considered in regulating the trade and in providing help to those who suffer from their own or other persons' gambling.

◆ The harm to society varies with the total amount of money and time spent on gambling. Game features and gambling environments have different potentials for harm and different capacities to collect money from players. The volume of the activity, game features, and gambling environments should be taken into consideration in policymaking.

◆ Simple prevalence measurements of problem gambling should be interpreted cautiously as indicators of the harm level and should not be used as the basis of policymaking. Variations in time may be especially misleading.

◆ The individuals counted in the small percentage of problem gamblers at any one time change from one period to the next, and the number of other persons affected by one problem gambler can be high. Policymakers should therefore guard against underestimating the dimensions of the problem in their societies.

◆ Effective techniques for preventing problem gambling include setting limits to: game intensity, inducements, and access to cash while gambling. By contrast, information, persuasion, self-assessment, and other personality-based responsible gambling tools have shown not to be effective.

◆ Effective pre-commitment and limit setting tools are those that are universally applied, mandatory, based on behavior, and implemented with personalized registration across the accessible forms of gambling participation.

◆ Government revenue and funding toward good causes from gambling create dependencies that may pressure policymaking. Gambling regulation should be separated from both of those interests.

• Regulation of online gambling is possible and is to be recommended as a harm-reduction policy.

• An international agreement on gambling control needs to be negotiated. The need for international control of online gambling makes this an urgent issue.

In conclusion, there is growing literature on effective policies and methods of prevention, and the evidence-base is sufficiently firm to ensure that their implementation has a high probability of success. The difficulty is political: the use of effective prevention measures will clash with other concerns, mostly financial. Efficient harm prevention requires compromise with these concerns, with a clear priority in favor of the public interest. The balance between the harm from gambling and the gains from it should not be sought by weighing the benefits and disadvantages of gambling to society as a whole. Instead, there should be analysis as to whether gambling is always the best way of achieving societal benefits, and whether the disadvantages could be addressed without increasing the burden on those already overburdened.

List of abbreviations and acronyms

ATM	Automated Teller Machine		**LDWs**	Losses Disguised as Wins
AUD	Australian Dollar		**NGO**	Nongovernmental Organization
CBA	Cost Benefit Analyses		**NOK**	Norwegian Kroner
CPGI	Canadian Problem Gambling Index		**NZD**	New Zealand Dollar
CSR	Corporate Social Responsibility		**OECD**	Organization for Economic Cooperation and Development
DNS	Domain Name System			
DSM	Diagnostic and Statistical Manual of the American Psychiatric Association		**PGSI**	Problem Gambling Severity Index
eCOGRA	E-Commerce and Online Gaming Regulation and Assurance		**PPGM**	Problem and Pathological Gambling Measure
			RTP ratio	Return to Player Ratio
EGM	Electronic Gambling Machine		**SOGS**	South Oaks Gambling Scale
EFTPOS	Electronic Fund Transfer Point of Sale		**TCM**	Total Consumption Model
			UIGEA	Unlawful Internet Gambling Enforcement Act
EU	European Union			
EUR	euros		**UK**	United Kingdom
GBP	Great Britain Pound		**UNESCO**	United Nations Educational, Scientific and Cultural Organization
GGR	Gross Gambling Revenue			
ICD	International Statistical Classification of Diseases and Related Health Problems of the World Health Organization		**UNODC**	United Nations Office on Drugs and Crime
			USD	United States Dollar
IGA	Interactive Gambling Act		**VLT**	Video Lottery Terminal
IGC	Interactive Gaming Council		**WHO**	World Health Organization
IP	Internet Protocol		**WTO**	World Trade Organization

References

Abait, P. E., & Folino, J. O. (2007). Characteristics of Pathological Gamblers in Argentina. *Vertex, 18*(75), 325–334.

Abbott, M. (2006). Do EGMs and Problem Gambling Go Together Like a Horse and Carriage? *Gambling Research, 18*(1), 7–38.

Abbott, M. W., Romild, U., & Volberg, R. A. (2014). Gambling and Problem Gambling in Sweden: Changes between 1998 and 2009. *Journal of Gambling Studies, 30*(4), 985–999.

Abbott, M., Stone, C.A., Billi, R., & Yeung, K. (2016). Gambling and Problem Gambling in Victoria, Australia: Changes over 5 years. *Journal of Gambling Studies, 32*(1), 47–78.

Abbott, M., & Volberg, R. (1992). *Frequent Gamblers and Problem Gamblers in New Zealand: Report on Phase Two of the National Survey*. Research Series, 14. Wellington: New Zealand Department of Internal Affairs.

Abbott, M. W., Volberg, R. A., & Rönnberg, S. (2004a). Comparing the New Zealand and Swedish National Surveys of Gambling and Problem Gambling. *Journal of Gambling Studies, 20*(3), 237–258.

Abbott, M. W., Williams, M. M., & Volberg, R. A. (2004b). A Prospective Study of Problem and Regular Nonproblem Gamblers Living in the Community. *Substance Use and Misuse, 39*(6), 855–884.

Abovitz, I. (2008). Why the United States Should Rethink its Legal Approach to Internet Gambling: A Comparative Analysis of Regulatory Models That Have Been Successfully Implemented in Foreign Jurisdictions. *Temple International and Comparative Law Journal, 22*, 437–470.

Adams, P. (2016). *Moral Jeopardy: Risks of Accepting Money from the Tobacco, Alcohol and Gambling Industries*. Cambridge: Cambridge University Press.

Adams, P. (2008). *Gambling, Freedom and Democracy*. New York: Routledge.

Adams, P. (2004). A History of Gambling in New Zealand. Guest Editorial to Special Issue. *Journal of Gambling Issues, 10*, 1–15.

Adams, P., Raeburn, J., & de Silva, K. (2009). A Question of Balance: Prioritizing Public Health Responses to Harm from Gambling. *Addiction, 104*(5), 688–691. doi: 10.1111/j.1360-0443.2008.02414.x

Ahmed, M. (2017). How UK Beat the Odds to Win at Online Gambling. *Financial Times* August, 12. https://www.ft.com/content/044a3d9e-7d1a-11e7-9108-edda0bcbc928

Alain, M. (2011). *The Establishment of the Trois-Rivieres Gaming Hall*. Trois-Rivieres: Universite du Quebec a Trois-Rivieres.

Albers, N., & Hübl, L. (1997). Gambling Market and Individual Patterns of Gambling in Germany. *Journal of Gambling Studies, 13*(2), 125–144.

American Psychiatric Association (2013). *Diagnostic and Statistical Manual of Mental Disorders* (5th edn). Arlington, VA: American Psychiatric Publishing.

Anderson, P. (2011). Gambling in Sports, in J. Naftziger & S. Ross, eds., *Handbook of International Sports Law*. Northampton, MA, USA: Edward Elgar Publishing, 162–207.

Anti-Mafia Commission. (2016). *Relazione Sulle Infiltrazioni Mafiose e Criminali Nel Gioco Lecito e Illecito* [Report on mafia and criminal infiltration into legal and illegal gambling]. Document XXIII No. 18, XVII Legislature.

Antonova, E. (2014). Vlasti Kryma Predlozhili Perenesti Igornuyu Zonu iz Yalty v Yevpatoriyu: http://top.rbc.ru/economics/12/11/2014/5463385fcbb20f0c73ca938d

Ariyabuddhiphongs, V. (2013). Adolescent Gambling: A Narrative Review of Behavior and its Predictors. *International Journal of Mental Health and Addiction*, *11*(1), 97–109.

ARJEL (Autorité de Régulation du Jeu en Ligne). 2015. *Rapport d'activité 2014–2015* [Annual Report 2014–2015]. Paris: ARJEL.

Audrain-McGovern, J., Rodriguez, D., Epstein, L. H., Cuevas, J., Rodgers, K., & Wileyto, E. P. (2009). Does Delay Discounting Play an Etiological Role in Smoking or is it a Consequence of Smoking? *Drug and Alcohol Dependence*, *103*(3), 99–106.

Auer, M., & Griffiths, M. (2014). Personalized Feedback in the Promotion of Responsible Gambling: A Brief Overview. *Responsible Gambling Review*, *1*(1), 27–36.

Auer, M., & Griffiths, M. (2013a). Voluntary Limit Setting and Player Choice in Most Intense Online Gamblers: An Empirical Study of Gambling Behaviour. *Journal of Gambling Studies*, *29*(4), 647–660. doi: 10.1007/s10899-012-9332-y

Auer M., & Griffiths M. (2013b). Behavioral Tracking Tools, Regulation, and Corporate Social Responsibility in Online Gambling. *Gaming Law Review: Economics, Regulation, Compliance, and Policy*, *17*(8), 579–583. https://doi.org/10.1089/glre.2013.1784

Auer, M., Malisching, D., & Griffiths, M. (2014). Is "Pop-Up" Messaging in Online Slot Machine Gambling Effective as a Responsible Gambling Strategy? *Journal of Gambling Issues*, *29*, 1–10. https://doi.org/10.4309/jgi.2014.29.3

Australian Gambling Statistics. (2016). *Australian Gambling Statistics 1989–90 to 2014–15 32nd edition*. Queensland Government Statistician's Office, Queensland Treasury.

Australian Institute for Gambling Research. (1995). *Report of the first year of the study into the social and economic impact of the introduction of gaming machines to Queensland clubs and hotels*. Brisbane, Australia: Queensland Department of Families, Youth and Community Care.

Australian Productivity Commission. (2010). *Inquiry Report—Gambling*. Report number 50, Australian Government.

Australian Productivity Commission. (1999). *Australia's Gambling Industries*. Final report. Summary. Report number 10, Australian Government.

Avtonomov, D. (2014). Issledovanie Obstoyatelstv Priobscheniya, Motivatsii i Otnosheniya K Ycastiyu V Azartnyh Igrah y Patsientov Na Raznyh Etapah Formirovaniya Zabisimosti [Investigation of the circumstances of initiation, motivation and attitudes to gambling in patients at different stages of dependency]. *Zhurnal Prakticeskoy Psihologii i Psihoanaliza, 3.*

Babor, T. F., Caetano, R., Casswell, S., Edwards, G., Giesbrecht, N., Graham, K., et al. (2010). *Alcohol: No Ordinary Commodity. Research and Public Policy* (2nd edn). Oxford: Oxford University Press.

Babor, T. F., & Del Boca, F. K. (2003). *Treatment Matching in Alcoholism*. Cambridge, UK: Cambridge University Press.

Babor, T. F., & Miller, P. (2014). McCarthyism, Conflict of Interest and Addiction's New Transparency Declaration Procedures. *Addiction, 109*, 341–344 [corrigendum 109:1389].

Babor, T. F., Morisano, D., Noel, J., Robaina, K., Ward, J. H., & Mitchell, A. L. (2017). Infrastructure and Career Opportunities in Addiction Science: The Emergence of an Interdisciplinary Field, in T. F. Babor et al. eds., *Publishing addiction science: A guide for the perplexed* (3rd edn). London: UK Ubiquity Press, 9–34.

Babor, T. F., Stenius, K., & Romelsjo, A. (2008). Alcohol and Drug Treatment Systems in Public Health Perspective: Mediators and Moderators of Population Effects. *International Journal of Methods in Psychiatric Research*, *17*(S1), 50–59.

Banks, J. (2014). *Online Gambling and Crime: Causes, Controls and Controversies*. Farnham: Ashgate Publishing.

Barclay, L. (2007). The Odds of Winning the National Lottery are 14 Million to One. Why Do People Play? http://tutor2u.net/blog/files/Louis_Barclay_Lottery.pdf

Barnard, M., Kerr, J., Kinsella, R., Orford, J., Reith, G., & Wardle, H. (2014). Exploring the Relationship Between Gambling, Debt and Financial Management in Britain. *International Gambling Studies*, *14*(1), 82–95.

Barnes, G. M., Welte, J. W., Tidwell, M. C. O., & Hoffman, J. H. (2015). Gambling and Substance Use: Co-occurrence Among Adults in a Recent General Population Study in the United States. *International Gambling Studies*, *15*(1), 55–71. http://dx.doi.org/10.1080/14459795.2014.990396

Barnes, G. M., Welte, J. W., Tidwell, M. C. O., & Hoffman, J. H. (2013). Effects of Neighborhood Disadvantage on Problem Gambling and Alcohol Abuse. *Journal of Behavioral Addictions*, *2*(2), 82–89. https://doi.org/10.1556/JBA.2.2013.004

Baron, E., & Dickerson, M. (1999). Alcohol Consumption and Self-Control of Gambling Behaviour. *Journal of Gambling Studies*, *15*(1), 3–15. doi: 10.1023/A:1023057027992

Barratt, M. J., Livingston, M., Matthews, S., & Clemens, S. L. (2014). Gaming Machine Density is Correlated with Rates of Help-Seeking for Problem Gambling: A Local Area Analysis in Victoria, Australia. *Journal of Gambling Issues*, *29*, 1–21. doi: https://doi.org/10.4309/jgi.2014.29.16

Barry, D., Pilver, C., Hoff, R., & Potenza, M. (2013). Pain Interference, Gambling Problem Severity, and Psychiatric Disorders Among a Nationally Representative Sample of Adults. *Journal of Behavioral Addictions*, *2*(3), 138–144. doi: https://doi.org/10.1556/JBA.2.2013.010

Baxandall, P., & Sacerdote, B. (2005). *Betting on the Future: The Economic Impact of Legalized Gambling*. Rappaport Institute for Greater Boston, Kennedy School of Government, Harvard University, # PB2005-1.

Beckert, J., & Lutter, M. (2013). Why the Poor Play the Lottery: Sociological Approaches to Explaining Class-Based Lottery Play. *Sociology*, *47*(6), 1152–1170.

Beckert, J., & Lutter, M. (2009). The Inequality of fair play: Lottery Gambling and Social Stratification in Germany. *European Sociological Review*, *25*(4), 475–488. doi: https://doi.org/10.1093/esr/jcn063

Bedford, K., Alvarez-Macotela, O., Casey, D., Kurban Jobin, M., & Williams, T. (2016). *The Bingo Project—Rethinking Gambling Regulation*. University of Kent: Economic and Social Research Council.

Beem, B., & Mikler, J. (2011). National Regulations for a Borderless Industry: US versus UK Approaches to Online Gambling. *Policy and Society*, *30*(3), 161–174. https://doi.org/10.1016/j.polsoc.2011.07.001

Beenstock, M., & Haitovsky, Y. (2001). Lottomania and Other Anomalies in the Market for Lotto. *Journal of Economic Psychology, 22*, 721–722. https://doi.org/10.1016/S0167-4870(01)00057-5

Bégin, C. (2001). *Pour une Politique des Jeux*. Paris: L'Harmattan.

Benegal, V. (2012). Gambling Experiences, Policy and Problems in India: A Historical Analysis. *Addiction, 108*, 2062–2067.

Betsson Group (2014). End of the Road for the Gaming Monopoly? Gaming Report 2014.

Binde, P. (2014). *Gambling Advertising: A Critical Research Review*. London: The Responsible Gambling Trust. http://hdl.handle.net/1880/51054

Binde, P. (2011). *What are the Most Harmful Forms of Gambling?* Analyzing Problem Gambling Prevalence Surveys. CEFOS Working Papers, 12. http://hdl.handle.net/2077/26165

Binde, P. (2009). Exploring the Impact of Gambling Advertising: An Interview Study of Problem Gamblers. *International Journal of Mental Health and Addiction, 7*(4), 541. doi: 10.1007/s11469-008-9186-9

Binde, P. (2007a). Gambling and Religion: Histories Of Concord And Conflict. *Journal of Gambling Issues, 20*, 145–165.

Binde, P. (2007b). Selling Dreams—Causing Nightmares? *Journal of Gambling Issues, 20*, 167–192.

Binde, P. (2005). Gambling Across Cultures: Mapping Worldwide Occurrence and Learning from Ethnographic Comparison. *International Gambling Studies, 5*(1), 1–27.

Black, D. W., Coryell, W., Crowe, R., McCormick, B., Shaw, M., & Allen, J. (2015). Suicide Ideations, Suicide Attempts, and Completed Suicide in Persons with Pathological Gambling and Their First-Degree Relatives. *Suicide and Life-threatening Behaviour, 45*(6), 700–709. doi: 10.1111/sltb.12162

Black, D. W., & Moyer, T. (1998). Clinical Features and Psychiatric Comorbidity of Subjects with Pathological Gambling Behavior. *Psychiatric Services, 49*(11), 1434–1439. https://doi.org/10.1176/ps.49.11.1434

Black, D. W., Shaw, M., McCormick, B., & Allen, J. (2013). Pathological Gambling: Relationship to Obesity, Self-Reported Chronic Medical Conditions, Poor Lifestyle Choices, and Impaired Quality of Life. *Comprehensive Psychiatry, 54*(2), 97–104. https://doi.org/10.1016/j.comppsych.2012.07.001

Black, D. W., Shaw, M. C., McCormick, B. A., & Allen, J. (2012). Marital Status, Childhood Maltreatment, and Family Dysfunction: A Controlled Study of Pathological Gambling. *Journal of Clinical Psychiatry, 73*(10), 1293. doi: 10.4088/JCP.12m07800

Blalock, G., Just, D. R., & Simon, D. H. (2007). Hitting the Jackpot or Hitting the Skids: Entertainment, Poverty, and the Demand for State Lotteries. *American Journal of Economics & Sociology, 66*(3), 545–570.

Bland, B. (2015). Profits at Macau's 6 Biggest Casino Operators Fall 40%. *Financial Times*, August 19. http://www.ft.com/intl/cms/s/0/668a56ae-463c-11e5-b3b2-1672f710807b.html#axzz42zOMN3Xi

Bland, R. C., Newman, S. C., Orn, H., & Stebelsky, G. (1993). Epidemiology of Pathological Gambling in Edmonton. *Canadian Journal of Psychiatry, 38*(2), 108–112.

Blaszczynski, A., Ladouceur, R., & Nower, L. (2007). Self-Exclusion: A Proposed Gateway to Treatment Model. *International Gambling Studies, 7*(1), 59–71. http://dx.doi.org/10.1080/14459790601157830

Blaszczynski, A., & Nower, L. (2002). A Pathways Model of Problem and Pathological Gambling. *Addiction*, *97*(5), 487–499. doi: 10.1046/j.1360-0443.2002.00015.x

Blaszczynski, A., Russell, A., Gainsburg, S., & Hing, N. (2016). Mental Health and Online, Land-Based and Mixed Gamblers. *Journal of Gambling Studies*, *32*(1), 261–275.

Blaszczynski, A., Sharpe, L., & Walker, M. (2001). *The Assessment of the Impact of the Reconfiguration on Electronic Gaming Machines as Harm Minimisation Strategies for Problem Gambling*: Final reports. The University of Sydney. http://www.psych.usyd.edu.au/gambling/GIO_report.pdf

Blaszczynski, A., & Silove, D. (1995). Cognitive and Behavioral Therapies for Pathological Gambling. *Journal of Gambling Studies*, *11*, 195–220.

Blinn-Pike, L., Worthy, S. L., & Jonkman, J. N. (2010). Adolescent Gambling: A Review of an Emerging Field of Research. *Journal of Adolescent Health*, *47*(3), 223–236. https://doi.org/10.1016/j.jadohealth.2010.05.003

Boardman, B., & Perry, J. J. (2007). Access to Gambling and Declaring Personal Bankruptcy. *Journal of Socio-Economics*, *36*(5), 789–801. https://doi.org/10.1016/j.socec.2007.01.012

Bol, T., Lancee, B., & Steijn, S. (2014). Income Inequality and Gambling: A Panel Study in the United States (1980–1997). *Sociological Spectrum*, *34*(1), 61–75. http://dx.doi.org/10.1080/02732173.2014.857196

Bondolfi, G., Jermann, F., Ferrero, F., Zullino, D., & Osiek, C. H. (2008). Prevalence of Pathological Gambling in Switzerland After the Opening of Casinos and the Introduction of New Preventive Legislation. *Acta Psychiatrica Scandinavica*, *117*(3), 236–239. doi: 10.1111/j.1600-0447.2007.01149.x

Borch, A. (2012). The Real of Problem Gambling Households. *Journal of Gambling Issues*, *27*. https://jgi.camh.net/index.php/jgi/article/viewFile/3866/3936

Bramley, S. (2015). *Exploring the Presence, Experience and Influence of Background Music in Gambling Situations*. PhD thesis, University of Sheffield.

Bramley, S., & Gainsbury, S. (2014). The Role of Auditory Features Within Slot-Themed Social Casino Games and Online Slot Machine Games. *Journal of Gambling Studies*, *31*(4), 1735–1751. doi: 10.1007/s10899-014-9506-x

Breen, B., Blaszczynski, A., & Anjoul, F. (2017). Systematic Review of Empirically Evaluated School-Based Gambling Education Programs. *Journal of Gambling Studies*, **33** (1), 301–325.

Breen, H. (2008). Visitors to Australia: Debating the History of Indigenous Gambling. *International Gambling Studies*, *8*(2), 137–150.

Breen, H., Hing, N., & Gordon, A. (2011). Indigenous Gambling Motivations, Behaviour and Consequences In Northern New South Wales, Australia. *International Journal of Mental Health and Addiction*, *9*(6), 723–739. doi: 10.1007/s11469-010-9293-2

Brenner, R., & Brenner, G. (1990). *Gambling and Speculation. A Theory, a History, and a Future for Some Human Decisions*. Cambridge: Cambridge University Press.

Brevers, D., Noël, X., Bechara, A., Vanavermaete, N., Verbanck, P., & Kornreich, C. (2015). Effect of Casino-Related Sound, Red Light and Pairs on Decision-Making During the Iowa Gambling Task. *Journal of Gambling Studies*, *31*(2), 409–421. doi: 10.1007/s10899-013-9441-2

Breyer, J. L., Botzet, A. M., Winters, K. C., Stinchfield, R. D., August, G., & Realmuto, G. (2009). Young Adult Gambling Behaviors and Their Relationship with the Persistence of ADHD. *Journal of Gambling Studies*, *25*(2), 227–238. doi: 10.1007/s10899-009-9126-z

Brezing, C., Derevensky, J. L., & Potenza, M. N. (2010). Non–Substance-Addictive Behaviors in Youth: Pathological Gambling and Problematic Internet Use. *Child and Adolescent Psychiatric Clinics of North America, 19*(3), 625–641.

Bridwell, R. R., & Quinn, F. L. (2002). From Mad Joy to Misfortune: The Merger of Law And Politics In The World Of Gambling. *Mississippi Law Journal, 72*(2), 565–729.

Broda, A., LaPlante, D., Nelson, S., LaBrie, R., Bosworth, L. & Shaffer, H. (2008). Virtual Harm Reduction Efforts for Internet Gambling: Effects of Deposit Limits on Actual Internet Sports Gambling Behavior. *Harm Reduction Journal, 5*(1), 27. doi: 10.1186/1477-7517-5-27

Brown, H. (2010). *A Review of Gambling-Related Issues*. City of Greater Dandenong. http://www.responsiblegambling.org.au/images/othersourcedocs/a-review-of-gambling-related-issues-2010%20hb%20cgd.pdf

Brown, S., Dickerson, A., McHardy, J., & Taylor, K. (2012). Gambling and Credit: An Individual and Household Level Analysis for the UK. *Applied Economics, 44*(35), 4639–4650.

Browne, A. (2015). China's Xi Jinping Changes the Odds in Macau. *The Wall Street Journal* October 1, 2015 http://www.wsj.com/articles/xi-changes-the-odds-in-macau-1444115241

Browne, B. R. (1991). The Selective Adaptation of the Alcoholics Anonymous Program by Gamblers Anonymous. *Journal of Gambling Studies, 7*(3), 187–206. doi: 10.1007/BF01019873

Browne, M., Langham, E., Rawat, V., Greer, N., Li, E., Rose, J., Rockloff, M., Donaldson, P., Thorne, H., Goodwin, B., Bryden, G., & Best, T. (2016). *Assessing Gambling-Related Harm in Victoria: A Public Health Perspective*. Victorian Responsible Gambling Foundation, Melbourne.

Browne, M., Greer, N, Armstrong, T, Doran, C, Kinchin, I, Langham, E & Rockloff, M. (2017). The social cost of gambling to Victoria, Victorian Responsible Gambling Foundation, Melbourne.

Bruun, K., Edwards, G., Lumio, M., Mäkelä, K., Pan, L., Popham, R. E., Room, R., Schmidt, W., Skog, O-J., Sulkunen, P., Österberg, E. (1975). *Alcohol Control Policies in Public Health Perspective*. Helsinki: The Finnish Foundation for Alcohol Studies Vol. **25**.

Bühringer, G., Braun, B., Kräplin, A., Neumann, M., Sleczka, P. (2013). *Gambling: Two Sides of the Same Coin*. AR Policy Brief 2. http://euspr.org/wp-content/uploads/2013/07/AR_PolicyPaper-2-Gambling_July-2013.pdf

Bullock, S., & Potenza, M. N. (2015). Pharmacological Treatments, in H. Bowden-Jones and S. George eds., *A Clinician's Guide to Working with Problem Gamblers*. Abingdon: Routledge, 134–162.

Caillois, R. (1958). *Les Jeux et les Hommes: Le Masque et le Vertige*. Paris: Gallimard.

Calado, F., Alexandre, J. & Griffiths, M. D. (2016). Prevalence of Adolescent Problem Gambling: A Systematic Review of Recent Research. *Journal of Gambling Studies, 33*(2), 397–424. doi: 10.1007/s10899-016-9627-5

Callan M. J., Ellard J. H., Shead N. W., & Hodgins D. C. (2008). Gambling as a Search for Justice: Examining the Role of Personal Relative Deprivation in Gambling Urges and Gambling Behavior. *Personality and Social Psychology Bulletin, 34*, 1514–1529. doi: 10.1177/0146167208322956

Callan, M. J., Shead, N. W., & Olson, J. M. (2011). Personal relative Deprivation, Delay Discounting, and Gambling. *Journal of Personality and Social Psychology, 101*, 955–973.

Campbell, C., Hartnagel, T., & Smith, G. (2005). The Legalization of Gambling in Canada. Ottawa, ON: A report prepared for the Law Commission of Canada.

Campbell, F., & Lester, D. (1999). The Impact of Gambling Opportunities on Compulsive Gambling. *Journal of Social Psychology, 139*(1), 126–127, doi: 10.1080/00224549909598366

Canu, W. H., & Schatz, N. K. (2011). A Weak Association Between Traits of Attention-Deficit/Hyperactivity Disorder and Gambling in College Students. *Journal of College Student Psychotherapy, 25*(4), 334–343. doi: http://dx.doi.org/10.1080/87568225.2011.605697

Carlton, P. L., Manowitz, P., McBride, H., Nora, R., Swartzburg, M., & Goldstein, L. (1987). Attention Deficit Disorder and Pathological Gambling. *Journal of Clinical Psychiatry, 48*(12), 487–488.

Carr, R. D., Buchkoski, J. E., Kofoed, L., & Morgan, T. J. (1996) "Video lottery" and Treatment for Pathological Gambling: A Natural Experiment in South Dakota. *South Dakota Journal of Medicine, 49*(1), 30–32.

Casey, L. M., Oei, T. P., Raylu, N., Horrigan, K., Day, J., Ireland, M., & Clough, B. A. (2017). Internet-Based Delivery of Cognitive Behaviour Therapy Compared to Monitoring, Feedback and Support for Problem Gambling: A Randomised Controlled Trial. *Journal of Gambling Studies*, 1–18. doi: 10.1007/s10899-016-9666-y

Cassidy, R., Loussouarn, C., & Pisac, A. (2013). *Fair Game: Producing Gambling Research.* The Goldsmiths Report.

Castrén, S., Basnet, S., Pankakoski, M., Ronkainen, J. E., Helakorpi, S., Uutela, A., & Lahti, T. (2013). An Analysis of Problem Gambling Among the Finnish Working-Age Population: A Population Survey. *BMC Public Health, 13*(1), 519. doi: 10.1186/1471-2458-13-519

Chamberlain, S. R., Derbyshire, K., Leppink, E., & Grant, J. E. (2015). Impact of ADHD Symptoms on Clinical and Cognitive Aspects of Problem Gambling. *Comprehensive Psychiatry, 57*, 51–57.

Chambers, K. (2011). *Gambling for Profit: Lotteries, Gaming Machines, and Casinos in Cross-National Focus.* Toronto: University of Toronto Press.

Chipman, M., Govoni, R., & Roerecke, M. (2006). *The Distribution of Consumption Model: An Evaluation of its Applicability to Gambling Behaviour.* Final report prepared for the Ontario Problem Gambling Research Centre.

Chóliz, M. (2016). The Challenge of Online Gambling: The Effect of Legalisation on the Increase in Online Gambling Addiction. *Journal of Gambling Studies, 32*(2), 749–756.

Chou, K. L., & Afifi, T. O. (2011). Disordered (Pathologic or Problem) Gambling and Axis I Psychiatric Disorders: Results from the National Epidemiologic Survey on Alcohol and Related Conditions. *American Journal of Epidemiology, 173*(11), 1289–1297.

Christie, S. (2017). Bet365 Chief Exec Denise Coates Becomes UK's Highest-Paid Boss After Earning £199m Last Year. *The Telegraph*, November, 13. http://www.telegraph.co.uk/business/2017/11/13/bet365-chief-exec-denise-coates-becomes-uks-highest-paid-boss/

Chun, J., Cho, S., Chung, I. J., & Kim, S. (2011). Economic and Psychosocial Impact of Problem Gambling in South Korea. *Asian Journal of Gambling Issues and Public Health, 2*(1), 29–38.

Cisneros Örnberg, J. C., & Tammi, T. (2011). Gambling Problems as a Political Framing—Safeguarding the Monopolies in Finland and Sweden. *Journal of Gambling Issues, 26*, 110–125. https://doi.org/10.4309/jgi.2011.26.8

Clark, C., Nower, L., & Walker, D. M. (2013). The Relationship of ADHD Symptoms to Gambling Behaviour in the USA: Results from the National Longitudinal Study of Adolescent Health. *International Gambling Studies*, *13*(1), 37–51. http://dx.doi.org/10.1080/14459795.2012.703213

Clark, L., Crooks, B., Clarke, R., Aitken, M., & Dunn, B. (2012). Physiological Responses to Near-Miss Outcomes and Personal Control During Simulated Gambling. *Journal of Gambling Studies*, *28*(1), 124–137. doi: 10.1007/s10899-011-9247-z

Clarke, D., Tse, S., Abbott, M., Townsend, S., Kingi, P., & Manaia, W. (2006). Key Indicators of the Transition from Social to Problem Gambling. *International Journal of Mental Health and Addiction*, *4*, 247–264.

Claybrook, J. (2007). Case Summary: WTO Internet Gambling Case. Public Citizen Online. March https://www.citizen.org/documents/Gamblingsummary2007.pdf

Clement, R., Goudriaan, A., van Holst, R., Molinaro, S., Moersen, C., Nilsson, T., Parke, A., Peren, F., Rebeggiani, L., Stoever, H., Terlau, W., & Wilheim, M. (2012). Measuring and Evaluating the Potential Addiction Risk of the Online Poker Game Texas Hold'em No Limit. *Gaming Law Review and Economics*, *16*(12), 713–728.

Clotfelter, C. T., & Cook, P. J. (1991). *Selling Hope: State Lotteries in America*. Cambridge, Mass.: Harvard University Press.

Clotfelter, C., Cook, P., Edell, J., & Moore, M. (1999). *State Lotteries at the Turn of the Century*. Report to the National Gambling Impact Study Commission.

Cook, S., Turner, N. E., Ballon, B., Paglia-Boak, A., Murray, R., Adlaf, E. M., & Mann, R. E. (2015). Problem Gambling Among Ontario Students: Associations with Substance Abuse, Mental Health Problems, Suicide Attempts, and Delinquent Behaviours. *Journal of Gambling Studies*, *31*(4), 1121–1134.

Copello, A., Templeton, L., Orford, J., & Velleman, R. (2010). The 5-Step Method: Evidence of Gains for Affected Family Members. *Drugs: Education, Prevention and Policy*, *17* (supl).

Corporate Research Associates (2006). *Nova Scotia Video Lottery Program Changes Impact Analysis*. Halifax: Nova Scotia Gaming Corporation.

Costes, J-M., Eroukmanoff, V., Richard, J-B., & Tovar, M-L. (2015). Les Jeux d'Argent et de Hasard en France en 2014 [Gambling in France in 2014]. *Les Notes de l'Observatoire des Jeux*, n° 6, 1–9.

Costes, J-M., Pousset, M., Eroukmanoff, V., Le Nezet, O., Richard, J. B., Guignard, R et al. (2011). *Les Niveaux et Pratiques des Jeux de Hazard et d'Argent en 2010* [The levels and practices of gambling in 2010]. OFDT, INPES, Paris: Tendances.

Côté, D., Caron, A., Aubert, J., Desrochers, V., & Ladouceur, R. (2003). Near Wins Prolong Gambling on a Video Lottery Terminal. *Journal of Gambling Studies*, *19*(4), 433–438. doi: 10.1023/A:1026384011003

Cour des Comptes (2016). *La Régulationd des Jeux d'Argent et de Hasard* [Regulation of gambling]. Comité d'évaluation de contrôle des politiques publiques de l'Assemblée nationale.

Cowlishaw, S., Merkouris, S., Chapman, A., & Radermacher, H. (2014). Pathological and Problem Gambling in Substance Use Treatment: A Systematic Review and Meta-Analysis. *Journal of Substance Abuse Treatment*, *46*(2), 98–105.

Cowlishaw, S., Merkouris, S., Dowling, N., Anderson, C., Jackson, A., & Thomas, S. (2012). *Psychological Therapies for Pathological and Problem Gambling*. The Cochrane Library. 10.1002/14651858.CD008937.pub2

Crane, M., Byrne, K., Fu, R., Lipmann, B., Mirabelli, F., Rota-Bartelink, A., et al. (2005). The Causes of Homelessness in Later Life: Findings from a 3-Nation Study. *Journal of Gerontology Social Sciences, 60B*(3), 152–159.

Crewe-Brown, C., Blaszczynski, A., & Russell, A. (2014). Prize Level and Debt Size: Impact on Gambling Behaviour. *Journal of Gambling Studies, 30*(3), 639–651. doi: 10.1007/s10899-013-9379-4

Croucher, J. S., Croucher, R. F., & Leslie, J. R. (2006). Report of the Pilot Study on the Self-Exclusion Program Conducted by GameChange (NSW).

Crowley, F., Eakins, J., & Jordan, D. (2013). Participation, Expenditure and Regressivity in the Irish lottery: Evidence from Irish Household Budget Survey 2004/2005. *The Economic and Social Review, 43*(2, Summer), 199–225.

Cunningham, J. A., Hodgins, D. C., Toneatto, T., & Murphy, M. (2012). A Randomized Controlled Trial of a Personalized Feedback Intervention for Problem Gamblers. *PLoS One, 7*(2), e31586. https://doi.org/10.1371/journal.pone.0031586

Cunningham, J. A., Hodgins, D. C., Toneatto, T., Rai, A., & Cordingley, J. (2009). Pilot Study of a Personalized Feedback Intervention for Problem Gamblers. *Behavior Therapy, 40*(3), 219–224. https://doi.org/10.1016/j.beth.2008.06.005

Cunningham-Williams, R. M., & Cottler, L. B. (2001). The Epidemiology of Pathological Gambling. *Seminars in Clinical Neuropsychiatry, 6*(3), 155–166.

Currie, S. R., Hodgins, D. C., Wang, J., El-Guebaly, N., Wynne, H., & Chen, S. (2006). Risk of Harm Among Gamblers in the General Population as a Function of Level of Participation in Gambling Activities. *Addiction, 101*(4), 570–580.

Currie, S. R., Hodgins, D. C., Wang, J., el-Guebaly, N., Wynne, H., & Miller, N. V. (2008). Replication of Low-Risk Gambling Limits Using Canadian Provincial Gambling Prevalence Data. *Journal of Gambling Studies, 24*(3), 321–335.

Dadayan, L. (2016). *State Revenues From Gambling: Short-Term Relief, Long-Term Disappointment. The Blinken Report.* New York: Rockefeller Institute.

Dadayan, L., Giguashvili, N., & Ward, R. B. (2008). *From a Bonanza to a Blue Chip? Gambling Revenues to the States.* Albany, NY: Rockefeller Institute Fiscal Features.

Dannon, P. N., Lowengrub, K., Aizer, A., & Kotler, M. (2006). Pathological Gambling: Comorbid Psychiatric Diagnoses in Patients and their Families. *Israel Journal of Psychiatry and Related Sciences, 43*(2), 88.

Darbyshire, P., Oster, C., & Carrig, H. (2001). The Experience of Pervasive Loss: Children and Young People Living in a Family where Parental Gambling is a Problem. *Journal of Gambling Studies, 17*(1), 23–45.

David, F. (1962). *Games, Gods and Gambling.* London: Charles Griffin and Co. Ltd.

Davis, D., Sundahl, I., & Lesbo, M. (2000). Illusory Personal Control as a Determinant of Bet Size and Type in Casino Raps Games. *Journal of Applied Social Psychology, 30*(6), 1224–1242. doi: 10.1111/j.1559-1816.2000.tb02518.x

Davis, R. (2006). All or Nothing: Video Lottery Terminal Gambling and Economic Restructuring in Rural Newfoundland. *Identities: Global Studies in Culture and Power, 13*(4), 503–531.

Debaise, C. (2011). Poker Crackdown: Time to Fold 'Em? *Wall Street Journal*, April 18, 2011. http://blogs.wsj.com/in-charge/2011/04/18/time-to-fold-em/

De Bruin, D. E., Benschop, A., Braam, R., & Korf, D. J. (2006). *Meerspelers: Meerjarige Monitor en Follow-Uponderzoek Naar Amusementscentra en Bezoekers* [Diverse gambling: Multiple year monitor and follow-up survey into amusement arcades and visitors]. Utrecht/Amsterdam: CVO/Bonger Instituut.

De Bruin, D. E., Leenders, F. R. J., Fris, M., Verbraeck, H. T., Braam, R. V., & van de Wijngaart, G. F. (2001). *Visitors of Holland Casino: Effectiveness of the Policy for the Prevention of Problem Gambling.* CVO University of Utrecht, the Netherlands: Addictions Research Institute.

De la Viña, L., & Bernstein, D. (2002). The Impact of Gambling on Personal Bankruptcy Rates. *Journal of Socio-Economics*, *31*(5), 503–509.

Delfabbro, P. (2013). Problem and Pathological Gambling: A Conceptual Review. *Journal of Gambling Business and Economics*, *7*(3), 35–53.

Delfabbro, P. (2009). *Australian Gambling Review* (4th edn). Adelaide: Independent Gambling Authority.

Delfabbro, P., Borgas, M., & King, D. (2012). Venue Staff Knowledge of their Patrons' Gambling and Problem Gambling. *Journal of Gambling Studies*, *28*(2), 155–169. doi: 10.1007/s10899-011-9252-2

Delfabbro, P., Falzon, K., & Ingram, T. (2005). The Effects of Parameter Variations in Electronic Gambling Simulations: Results of a Laboratory-Based Pilot Investigation. *Gambling Research*, *17*(1), 7–25.

Delfabbro, P., King, D., & Griffiths, M. D. (2014). From Adolescent to Adult Gambling: An Analysis of Longitudinal Gambling Patterns in South Australia. *Journal of Gambling Studies*, *30*(3), 547–563.

Delfabbro, P., Osborn, A., Nevile, M., Skelt, L., & McMillen, J. (2007). *Identifying Problem Gamblers in Gambling Venues: Final Report.* Report commissioned for the Ministerial Council on Gambling. Melbourne, Victoria, Australia.

Delfabbro, P., & Winefield, A. (1999). Pokermachine Gambling: An Analysis of Within Session Characteristics. *British Journal of Psychology*, *90*(3), 425–439.

Delfabbro, P., Winefield, A., & Anderson, S. (2009). Once a Gambler, Always a Gambler? A Longitudinal Analysis of Gambling Patterns in Young People Making the Transition From Adolescence to Adulthood. *International Gambling Sudies*, *9*(2), 151–163.

Derevensky, J. & Gupta, R. (2000). Youth Gambling: A Clinical and Research Perspective. *Journal of Gambling Issues, 2.*

Derevensky, J., Gupta, R., Messerlian, C., & Mansour, S. (2009). The Impact of Gambling Advertisement on Child and Adolescent Behaviors: A Qualitative Analysis. McGill University.

Derevensky, J. L., Gupta, R., & Winters, K. (2003). Prevalence Rates of Youth Gambling Problems: Are the Current Rates Inflated? *Journal of Gambling Studies*, *19*(4), 405–425.

Desai, R. A. & Potenza, M. N. (2009). A Cross-Sectional Study of Problem and Pathological Gambling in Patients with Schizophrenia/Schizoaffective Disorder. *Journal of Clinical Psychiatry*, *70*(9), 1250–1257.

Descotils, Gérard & Guilbert, J-C. (1993). *Le Grand Livre Des Loteries—Histoire Des Jeux de Hasard en France.* Paris: La Française des Jeux.

Di Nicola, M., De Risio, L., Pettorruso, M., Caselli, G., De Crescenzo, F., Swierkosz-Lenart, K., & Janiri, L. (2014). Bipolar Disorder and Gambling Disorder Comorbidity: Current Evidence and Implications for Pharmacological Treatment. *Journal of Affective Disorders*, *167*, 285–298.

Dixon, M. J., Fugelsang, J. A., MacLaren, V. V., & Harrigan, K. A. (2013). Gamblers Can Discriminate "Tight"From "Loose"Electronic Gambling Machines. *International Gambling Studies, 13*(1), 98–111.

Dixon, M., Harrigan, K., Santesso, D., Graydon, C., Fugelsang, J., & Collins, K. (2014). The Impact of Sound in Modern Multiline Video Slot Machine Play, *Journal of Gambling Studies, 30*(4), 913–929. doi: 10.1007/s10899-013-9391-8

Dowling, N. (2014). *The Impact of Gambling Problems on Families.* Australian Gambling Research Centre, Australian Institute of Family Studies. Final Report. https://aifs.gov.au/agrc/sites/default/files/publication-documents/agrc-dp1-family-impacts_0.pdf

Dowling, N., Jackson, A., Thomas, S., & Frydenberg, E. (2010). *Children at Risk of Developing Problem Gambling. Melbourne*: Gambling Research Australia. http://www.jogoremoto.pt/docs/extra/1HISat.pdf

Dowling, N., Rodda, S. N., Lubman, D. I., & Jackson, A. C. (2014). The Impacts of Problem Gambling on Concerned Significant Others Accessing Web-Based Couselling. *Addictive Behaviors, 39*(8), 1253–7.

Dowling N, Smith D, Thomas T. (2005). Electronic Gaming Machines: Are they the 'Crack-Cocaine' Of Gambling? *Addiction, 100*(1), 33–45.

Dowling, N., Suomi, A., Jackson, A., Lavis, T., Patford, J., Cockman, S., Thomas, S., Bellringer, M., Koziol-Mclain, J., Battersby, M., Harvey, P., & Abbott, M. (2016). Problem Gambling and Intimate Partner Violence. A Systematic Review and Meta-Analysis, *Trauma Violence Abuse, 17*(1), 43–61.

Downs, C., & Woolrych, R. (2010). Gambling and Debt: The Hidden Impacts on Family and Work Life. *Community, Work and Family, 13*(3), 311–328.

Downs, C., & Woolrych, R. (2009). *Gambling and Debt Pathfinder Study. Final Report,* 173.

Drakeford, B., & Hudson Smith, M. (2015). Mobile Gambling: Implications for Accessibility. *Journal of Research Studies in Business & Management 1*(1), 3–28.

Dufour, J., Ladouceur, R., & Giroux, I. (2010). Training Program on Responsible Gambling Among Video Lottery Employees. *International Gambling Studies, 10*(1), 61–79. http://dx.doi.org/10.1080/14459791003743037

Dufour, M., Roy, E., Boivin, J. F., Boudreau, J. F., & Robert, M. (2014). Correlates of At-risk Gambling Behaviors of Homeless Youth. *Journal of Addiction Research & Therapy,* 1–8. doi: 10.4172/2155-6105.S10-007

Duran, R. (2013). Gambling in Brazil. The Brazil Business, October 7, 2013. Online. http://thebrazilbusiness.com/article/gambling-in-brazil

Dunstan, R. (1997). *Gambling in California.* California Research Bureau, California State Library.

Durdle, H., Gorey, K. M., & Stewart, S. H. (2008). A Meta-Analysis Examining the Relations Among Pathological Gambling, Obsessive-Compulsive Disorder, and Obsessive-Compulsive Traits 1, 2. *Psychological Reports, 103*(2), 485–498.

Dzik, B. (2009). Poland, in G. Meyer et al. eds., *Problem Gambling in Europe: Challenges, Prevention, and Interventions.* New York: Springer.

Eadington, W. R. (1999). The Economics of Casino Gaming. *Journal of Economic Perspectives, 13*(3), 173–192.

Eby, L. T., Mitchell, M. E., Gray, C. J., Provolt, L., Lorys, A., Fortune, E., & Goodie, A. S. (2016). Gambling-Related Problems Across Life Domains: An Exploratory Study of Non-Treatment-Seeking Weekly Gamblers. *Community, Work & Family, 19*(5), 604–620.

Economist, The (2017). *The World's Biggest Gamblers*. The Data Team of The Economist, February, 9. http://www.economist.com/blogs/graphicdetail/2017/02/daily-chart-4

Edwards, G., Anderson, P., Babor, T., Casswell, S., Ferrence, R. Giesbrecht, N., Godfrey, C., Holder, H., & Lemmens, P. (1994). *Alcohol Policy and the Public Good*. Oxford: Oxford University Press.

EGBA European Gaming & Betting Association (2016). *Market Realty*. http://www.egba.eu/media/FACTSHEET_MARKET-REALITY3.pdf

Egerer, M., Hellman, M., Rolando, S., & Bujalski, M. (2016). Positions on Problematic Gambling by General Practitioners' in Three European Welfare States, in M. Hellman, V. Berridge, K. Duke, & A. Mold eds., *Concepts of Addictive Substances and Behaviours across Time and Place*. Oxford: Oxford University Press.

Egerer, M., Marionneau, V., & Nikkinen, J. eds. (2018 forthcoming). *Gambling Policies in European Welfare States—Current Challenges and Future Prospects*. London: Palgrave Macmillan.

Eimer, D. (2010). China's Secret Gambling Problem. *Telegraph* January 9, 2010. Online. http://www.telegraph.co.uk/news/worldnews/asia/china/6942975/Chinas-secret-gambling-problem.html

el-Guebaly, N., Patten, S. B., Currie S., Williams, J. V. A., Beck, C. A., Maxwell C. J., & Wang J. L. (2006). Epidemiological Associations Between Gambling Behavior, Substance Use & Mood and Anxiety Disorders. *Journal of Gambling Studies*, *22*(3), 275–287.

Ellery, M., & Stewart, S. H. (2014). Alcohol Affects Video Lottery Terminal (VLT) Gambling Behaviors and Cognitions Differently. *Psychology of Addictive Behaviors*, *28*(1), 206–216. http://dx.doi.org/10.1037/a0035235

Ellery, M., Stewart, S. H., & Loba, P. (2005). Alcohol Effects on Video Lottery Terminal (VLT) Play Among Probable Pathological and Non-Pathological Gamblers. *Journal of Gambling Studies*, *21*(3), 299–324. doi: 10.1007/s10899-005-3101-0

Engebø, J. & F. Gyllstrøm (2008). Regulatory Changes and Finally a Ban on Existing Slot Machines in Norway: What's the Impact on the Market and Problem Gambling? Presented at the 2008 International Gambling Conference. Auckland, New Zealand, February 2008.

European Commission (2012). *Online Gambling in the Internal Market*. Commission Staff Working Document. http://eur-lex.europa.eu/legal-content/EN/TXT/?uri=CELEX:52012SC0345

Evans, W., & Topoleski, J. (2002). *The Social and Economic Impact of Native American Casinos*. NBER Working Paper 9198. doi: 10.3386/w9198

Fahrenkopf, F. (2012). Introduction, in J. Harris ed. *Gaming Law. Jurisdictional Comparisons*. European Lawyer Reference Series (1st edn). London: Thomson Reuters, vii–xi.

FATF (Financial Action Task Force)/OECD (2009). Money Laundering Through the Football Sector. July 2009. http://www.fatf-gafi.org/media/fatf/documents/reports/ML%20through%20the%20Football%20Sector.pdf

Fekjær H. (2008). *Spilleavhengighet: Vår Nye Landeplage* [Gambling addiction: Our new scourge]. Oslo: Gyldendal Akademisk.

Felsher, J. R., Derevensky, J. L., & Gupta, R. (2003). Parental Influences and Social Modelling of Youth Lottery Participation. *Journal of Community & Applied Social Psychology*, *13*(5), 361–377.

Ferentzy, P. & Turner, N. (2013). *The History of Problem Gambling: Temperance, Substance Abuse, Medicine, and Metaphors*. New York: Springer.

Ferentzy, P., & Turner, N. (2009). Gambling and Organized Crime: A Review of the Literature. *Journal of Gambling Issues, 23,* 111–155.

Ferland, F., Fournier, P. M., Ladouceur, R., Brochu, P., Bouchard, M., & Pâquet, L. (2008). Consequences Of Pathological Gambling on the Gambler and his Spouse. *Journal of Gambling Issues, 22,* 219–229.

Ferris, J., & Wynne, H. (2001). *The Canadian Problem Gambling Index*. Ottawa, ON: Canadian Centre on Substance Abuse.

Fiedler, I. (2016a). *Glücksspiele. Eine verhaltens- und gesundheitsökonomische Analyse mit rechtspolitischen Empfehlungen*. Frankfut/M: Peter Lang.

Fiedler, I. (2016b). Möglichkeiten und Herausforderungen bei der Blockierung von Zahlungsströmen im Internet. Presentation at the Symposium Glücksspiel 2016, Universität Hohenheim (Germany).

Finlay, K., Marmurek, H., Kanetkar, V., & Londerville, J. (2010). Casino Décor Effects on Gambling Emotions and Intentions. *Environment & Behavior, 42* (4), 524–545.

Finlay, K., Marmurek, H. H. C., Kanetkar, V., & Londerville, J. (2007). Trait and State Emotion Congruence in Simulated Casinos: Effects on At-Risk Gambling Intention and Restoration. *Journal of Environmental Psychology, 27*(2), 166–175. https://doi.org/10.1016/j.jenvp.2007.03.002

Fisher, D. (2013). Facial Recognition Technology to Nab Casino's Banned Gamblers, *New Zealand Herald*, June, 25. https://www.nzherald.co.nz/nz/news/article.cfm?c_id=1&objectid=10892751

Foderaro, L. (2016). A Connecticut Tribe Fights for Recognition, and for Piece of Casino Industry, *New York Times*, June 27. https://www.nytimes.com/2016/06/28/nyregion/schaghticoke-tribe-connecticut-fights-for-piece-of-casino-industry.html

Forsström, D., Hesser, H., & Carlbring, P. (2016). Usage of A Responsible Gambling Tool: A Descriptive Analysis and Latent Class Analysis of User Behaviour. *Journal of Gambling Studies, 32*(3), 889–904. doi: 10.1007/s10899-015-9590-6

Frahn, T., Delfabbro, P., & King, D. (2015). Exposure to Free-Play Modes in Simulated Online Gaming Increases Risk-Taking in Monetary Gambling. *Journal of Gambling Studies, 31* (4), 1531–1543. doi: 10.1007/s10899-014-9479-9

French, M. T., Maclean, J. C., & Ettner, S. L. (2008). Drinkers and Bettors: Investigating the Complementarity of Alcohol Consumption and Problem Gambling. *Drug and Alcohol Dependence, 96*(1), 155–164.

Freund, E. & Morris, I. (2006). Gambling and Income Inequality in the States. *Policy Studies Journal, 34*(2), 265–276.

Freund, E. & Morris, I. (2005). The Lottery and Income Inequality in the States. *Social Science Quarterly, 86*(S1), 996–1012.

Friend, K. B., & Ladd, G. T. (2009). Youth Gambling Advertising: A Review of the Lessons Learned from Tobacco Control. *Drugs: Education, prevention and policy, 16*(4), 283–297. http://dx.doi.org/10.1080/09687630701838026

Frisch, G. R. (1999). *Community Impact of Increased Gambling Availability on Adult Gamblers—A Four Year Follow-Up*. Windsor, Ontario: Problem Gambling Group, University of Windsor.

Fromson, B. D. (2004). *Hitting the Jackpot: The Inside Story of The Richest Indian Tribe In History.* Atlantic Monthly Press.

Fulton, C. (2015). *Playing Social Roulette: The Impact of Gambling on Individuals and Society in Ireland.* University College Dublin.

Gainsbury, S. (2014). Review of Self-Exclusion from Gambling Venues as an Intervention for Problem Gambling. *Journal of Gambling Studies, 30*(2), 229–251. https://link. springer.com/article/10.1007/s10899-013-9362-0

Gainsbury, S. (2012). *Internet Gambling: Current Research Findings and Implications.* New York: Springer-Verlag.

Gainsbury, S., Aro, D., Ball, D., Tobar, C., & Russell, A. (2015). Optimal Content for Warning Messages to Enhance Consumer Decision Making and Reduce Problem Gambling. *Journal of Business Research, 68*(10), 2093–2101. https://doi.org/10.1016/j.jbusres.2015.03.007

Gainsbury, S., Russell, A., Hing, N., Wood, R., Lubman, D. & Blaszczynski, A., (2014b). The Prevalence and Determinants of Problem Gambling in Australia: Assessing the Impact of Interactive Gambling and New Technologies. *Psychology of Addictive Behaviors, 28*(3), 769–779.

Gainsbury, S., & Wood, R. (2011). Internet Gambling Policy in Critical Comparative Perspective: The Effectiveness of Existing Regulatory Frameworks. *International Gambling Studies, 11*(3), 309–323. http://dx.doi.org/10.1080/14459795.2011.619553

Gallet, C. A. (2015). Gambling Demand: A Meta-Analysis of the Price Elasticity. *Journal of Gambling Business and Economics, 9*(1), 12–22.

Gambling Commission UK (May/November) Industry statistics http://www. gamblingcommission.gov.uk/news-action-and-statistics/Statistics-and-research/ Statistics/Industry-statistics.aspx

Gandolfo, A., & De Bonis, V. (2013). Il Modello Italiano di Tassazione del Gioco D'azzardo: Linee Guida di Politica Fiscale per lo 'Sviluppo Sostenibile di un Mercato Importante e Controverso [The Italian gambling taxation system: Guidelines of fiscal policy for a sustainable development of an important and controversial market]. *Discussion Papers of the Economy and Management Department—Università di Pisa,* n. 173 https://www.ec.unipi.it/documents/Ricerca/papers/2013-173.pdf

Gattis, M., & Cunningham-Williams, R. (2011). Housing Stability and Problem Gambling: Is there a Relationship? *Journal of Social Service Research, 37*(5), 490–499.

George, S., & Bowden-Jones, H. (2015). Family Interventions in Gambling, in H. Bowden-Jones & S. George eds., *A Clinician's Guide to Working with Problem Gamblers.* New York: Routledge, 163–171.

Gerstein, D. R., Volberg, R. A., Toce, M. T., Harwood, H., Palmer, A., Johnson, R., Larison, C., Chuchro, L., Buie, T., Engelman, L. & Hill, M.A. (1999). *Gambling Impact and Behavior Study: Report to the National Gambling Impact Study Commission.* Chicago, IL: National Opinion Research Center at the University of Chicago.

Giddens, J. L., Xian, H., Scherrer, J. F., Eisen, S. A., & Potenza, M. N. (2011). Shared Genetic Contributions to Anxiety Disorders and Pathological Gambling in a Male Population. *Journal of Affective Disorders, 132*(3), 406–412.

Gidluck, L. (2016). A Global Comparison of how Governments Regulate, Operate and Benefit from State Lotteries. All Bets Are Off Conference, Canterbury, UK, June 24, 2016.

Gifford, E. V., Ritsher, J. B., McKellar, J. D., & Moos, R. H. (2006). Acceptance and Relationship Context: A Model of Substance Use Disorder Treatment Outcome. *Addiction, 101*(8), 1167–1177. doi: 10.1111/j.1360-0443.2006.01506.x

Giles, C. (2000). In Spain, Blind Lead the Blind—for Better. *Los Angeles Times,* July 2, 2000. http://articles.latimes.com/2000/jul/02/news/mn-46882

Gilliland, J. A., & Ross, N. A. (2005). Opportunities for Video Lottery Terminal Gambling in Montréal: An Environmental Analysis. *Canadian Journal of Public Health/Revue Canadienne de Santée Publique, 96*(1), 55–59.

Gmel, G., & Rehm, J. (2004). Measuring Alcohol Consumption. *Contemporary Drug Problems, 31*(3), 467–540.

Goss, E. P., & Morse, E. A. (2009). *Governing Fortune: Casino Gambling in America.* University of Michigan Press, 77–79.

Goss, E., & Morse, E. (2005). The Impact of Casino Gambling on Individual Bankruptcy Rates from 1990 to 2002, Creighton University: Working Paper.

Götestam, K. G., & Johansson, A. (2009). Norway, in G. Meyer et al. eds., *Problem Gambling in Europe: Challenges, Prevention, and Interventions.* New York: Springer.

Goudriaan, A. E. (2014). Gambling and Problem Gambling in the Netherlands. *Addiction 109*(7), 1066–1071.

Govoni, R. J. (2000). Gambling Behavior and the Distribution of Alcohol Consumption Model. Electronic Theses and Dissertations. Paper 2186. Windsor: University of Windsor.

Govoni, R., Frisch, G. R., Rupcich, N., & Getty, H. (1998). First Year Impacts of Casino Gambling in a Community. *Journal of Gambling Studies, 14*(4), 347–358.

Grant, D. (1994). *On a Roll: A History of Gambling and Lotteries in New Zealand.* Wellington: Victoria University Press.

Grant, J. E., Desai, R. A., & Potenza, M. N. (2009). Relationship of Nicotine Dependence, Subsyndromal and Pathological Gambling, and Other Psychiatric Disorders: Data from the National Epidemiologic Survey on Alcohol and Related Conditions. *Journal of Clinical Psychiatry, 70*(3), 334.

Grant, J. E., Kushner, M. G., & Kim, S. W. (2002). Pathological Gambling and Alcohol Use Disorder. *Alcohol Research and Health, 26*(2), 143–150.

Grant, J. E., Schreiber, L., Odlaug, B. L., & Kim, S. W. (2010). Pathologic Gambling and Bankruptcy. *Comprehensive psychiatry, 51*(2), 115–120.

Griffiths, M. (2010). Crime and Gambling: A Brief Overview Of Gambling Fraud on the Internet. *Internet Journal of Criminology,* 1–7. http://irep.ntu.ac.uk/id/eprint/23349/

Griffiths, M. (2009). Internet Gambling in the Workplace. *Journal of Workplace Learning, 21*(8), 658–670.

Griffiths, M. (2005). Structural Characteristics of Video Lotteries: Effects of a Stopping Device on Illusion of Control and Gambling Persistence. *Journal of Gambling Studies, 21*(2), 117–131. doi: 10.1007/s10899-005-3028-5

Griffiths, M. (1993). Fruit Machine Gambling: The Importance of Structural Characteristics. *Journal of Gambling Studies, 9*(2),101–120. doi: 10.1007/BF01014863

Griffiths, M., Scarfe, A., & Bellringer, P. (1999). The UK National Telephone Gambling Helpline—Results on the First Year of Operation. *Journal of Gambling Studies, 15*(1), 83–90. doi: 10.1023/A:1023071113879

Griffiths, M., & Parke, J. (2005). The Psychology of Music in Gambling Environments: An Observational Research Note. *Journal of Gambling Issues, 13.* https://doi.org/10.4309/jgi.2005.13.8

Griffiths, M., Wardle, H., Orford, J., Sproston, K., & Erens, B. (2009a). Sociodemographic Correlates of Internet Gambling: Findings from the 2007 British Gambling Prevalence Survey. *CyberPsychology & Behavior, 12*(2), 199–202.

Griffiths, M., & Wood, R. (2001). The Psychology of Lottery Gambling. *International Gambling Studies, 1*(1), 27–45. http://dx.doi.org/10.1080/14459800108732286

Griffiths, M., Wood, R., & Parke, J. (2009b). Social Responsibility Tools in Online Gambling: A Survey of Attitudes and Behaviour Among Internet Gamblers. *Cyber Psychology & Behavior, 12*(4), 413–421. https://doi.org/10.1089/cpb.2009.0062

Grinols, E., & Mustard, D. (2006). Casinos, Crime and Community Costs. *The Review of Economics and Statistics, 88*(1), 28–45.

Grote, K., & Matheson, V. (2011). The Economics of Lotteries: A Survey of the Literature. *Economics Department Working Papers. Paper 16.* http://crossworks.holycross.edu/econ_working_papers/16

Grun, L., & McKeigue, P. (2000). Prevalence of Excessive Gambling Before and After Introduction of a National Lottery in the United Kingdom: Another Example of the Single Distribution Theory. *Addiction, 95*(6), 959–966.

Guardian, The (2014). *Ndrangheta mafia 'made more last year than McDonald's and Deutsche Bank'* March, 26 https://www.theguardian.com/world/2014/mar/26/ndrangheta-mafia-mcdonalds-deutsche-bank-study

Guttentag, D., Harrigan, K., & Smith, S. (2012). Gambling by Ontario Casino Employees: Gambling Behaviours, Problem Gambling and Impacts of the Employment. *International Gambling Studies, 12*(1), 5–22.

Haefeli, J., & Lischer, S. (2010). Die Früherkennung von Problemspielern in Schweizer Kasinos. *Prävention und Gesundheitsförderung, 5*(2), 145–150. doi: 10.1007/s11553-009-0213-x

Haefeli, J., Lischer, S., & Schwartz, J. (2011). Early Detection Items and Responsible Gambling Features for Online Gambling. *Internet Gambling, 11*(3), 273–288. http://dx.doi.org/10.1080/14459795.2011.604643

Hansen, M., & Rossow, I. M. (2012). Does a Reduction in the Overall Amount of Gambling Imply a Reduction At All Levels of Gambling? *Addiction Research & Theory, 20*(2), 145–152.

Hansen, M., & Rossow, I. (2010). Limited Cash Flow on Slot Machines: Effects of Prohibition of Note Acceptors on Adolescent Gambling Behaviour. *International Journal of Mental Health and Addiction, 8*(1), 70–81. doi: 10.1007/s11469-009-9196-2

Hansen, M., & Rossow, I. (2008). Adolescent Gambling and Problem Gambling: Does the Total Consumption Model Apply? *Journal of Gambling Studies, 24*(2), 135–149.

Hare, S. (2015). *Study of Gambling and Health in Victoria.* Melbourne: Victorian Responsible Gambling Foundation.

Hare, S. (2009). *A Study of Gambling in Victoria: Problem Gambling from a Public Health Perspective.* Melbourne: Department of Justice.

Harrigan, K., Dixon, M., MacLaren, V., Collins, K., & Fugelsang, J. (2011). The Maximum Rewards at the Minimum Price: Reinforcement Rates and Payback Percentages in

Multi-Line Slot Machines. *Journal of Gambling Issues*, *26*, 11–29. https://doi.org/10.4309/jgi.2011.26.3

Harrigan, K., & MacLaren, V. (2014). *The House Rules: Gaming Regulations and their Effects on Gambling and Problem Gambling Across Canada*. University of Waterloo: Research Report for the Ontario Problem Gambling Research Centre.

Harrigan, K., MacLaren, V., Brown, D., Dixon, M. J., & Livingstone, C. (2014). Games of Chance or Masters of Illusion: Multiline Slots Design May Promote Cognitive Distortions. *International Gambling Studies*, *14*(2), 301–317.

Harrigan, K., MacLaren, V., & Dixon, M. (2010). *Effectiveness of a Brief Educational Intervention and ATM-Removal in Reducing Erroneous Cognitions and Over-Expenditure During Slot Machine Play in Problem and Non-Problem Gamblers*. Report to the Ontario Problem Gambling Research Centre.

Harris, A. & Parke, A. (2015). Empirical Evidence for the Differential Impact of Gambling Outcome on Behaviour in Electronic Gambling: Implications for Harm-Minimisation Strategies. *Responsible Gambling Review*, *1*(2), 10–19. http://eprints.lincoln.ac.uk/17024/

Harvey, M., Finlay, K., Kanetkar, V., & Londerville, J. (2007). The Influence of Music on Estimates of At-Risk Gambling Intentions: An Analysis by Casino Design. *International Gambling Studies*, *7*(1), 113–122. http://dx.doi.org/10.1080/14459790601158002

Haworth, L. (2008). Russian Roulette? Gambling in the Post-Soviet Era. *Gaming Law Review and Economics*, *12*(5), 466–469.

Haydock, M., Cowlishaw S., Harvey C., & Castle D. (2015). Prevalence and Correlates of Problem Gambling in People with Psychotic Disorders. *Comprehensive Psychiatry*, *58*, 122–129.

Hayer, T., & Meyer, G. (2011a). Self-Exclusion as a Harm Minimization Strategy: Evidence from the Casino Sector from Selected European Countries. *Journal of Gambling Studies*, *27*(4), 685–700. doi: 10.1007/s10899-010-9227-8

Hayer, T., & Meyer, G. (2011b). Internet Self-Exclusion: Characteristics of Self-Excluded Gamblers and Preliminary Evidence for its Effectiveness. *International Journal of Mental Health and Addiction*, *9*(3), 307–596. doi: 10.1007/s11469-010-9288-z

Hayer, T. & Meyer, G. (2005). *The Addictive Potential of Sports Betting. Empirical Data from a German Treatment-Seeking Population*. Presentation. European Association for the Study of Gambling, 6th European Conference on Gambling Studies and Policy Issues. http://gerhard.meyer.uni-bremen.de/index_dateien/Malm%F6_Hayer.pdf

Hing, N. (2003). *An Assessment of Member Awareness, Perceived Adequacy and Perceived Effectiveness of Responsible Gambling Strategies in Sydney Clubs*. Southern Cross University ePublications, http://epubs.scu.edu.au/cgi/viewcontent.cgi?article=1477&context=tourism_pubs

Hing, N. & Breen, H. (2008). How Working in a Gaming Venue Can Lead to Problem Gambling: The Experiences of Six Gaming Venue Staff. *Journal of Gambling Issues*, *21*, 11–29.

Hing, N., & Haw, J. (2010). *The Influence of Venue Characteristics on a Player's Decision to Attend a Gambling Venue*. Centre for Gambling Education and Research. http://www.researchgate.net/profile/Nerilee_Hing/publication/49403727_Influence_of_venue_characteristics_on_a_player's_decision_to_attend_a_gambling_venue/links/02e7e51ccd033e518a000000.pdf

Hing, N., & Nuske, E. (2012). Responding to Problem Gamblers in the Venue: Role Conflict, Role Ambiguity, and Challenges for Hospitality Staff. *Journal of Human Resources in Hospitality & Tourism*, *11*(2), 146–164. http://dx.doi.org/10.1080/15332845.2012.648896

Hing, N., & Nuske, E. (2011). Assisting Problem Gamblers in the Gaming Venue: An Assessment of Practices and Procedures Followed by Frontline Hospitality Staff. *International Journal of Hospitality Management*, *30*(2), 459–467. https://doi.org/10.1016/j.ijhm.2010.09.013

Hing, N., Russell, A., Tolchard, B., & Nower, L. (2016). Risk Factors for Gambling Problems: An Analysis by Gender. *Journal of Gambling Studies*, *32*(2), 511–534.

Hing, N., Tiyce, M., Holdsworth, L., & Nuske, E. (2013). All in the Family: Help-Seeking by Significant Others of Problem Gamblers. *International Journal of Mental Health and Addiction*, *11*(3), 396–408.

Hodgins, D., Currie, S. R., & el-Guebaly, N. (2001). Motivational Enhancement and Self-Help Treatments for Problem Gambling. *Journal of Consulting and Clinical Psychology*, *69*(1), 50–57. http://dx.doi.org/10.1037/0022-006X.69.1.50

Hodgins, D., Currie, S., el-Guebaly, N., Peden, N. (2004). Brief Motivational Treatment for Problem Gambling: A 24-Month Follow-Up. *Psychology of Addictive Behaviors*, *18*(3), 2004, 293–296. http://dx.doi.org/10.1037/0893-164X.18.3.293

Hodgins, D., & el-Guebaly, N. (2010). The Influence of Substance Dependence and Mood Disorders on Outcome from Pathological Gambling: Five-Year Follow-Up. *Journal of Gambling Studies*, *26*(1), 117–127.

Hodgins, D. & el-Guebaly, N. (2004). Retrospective and Prospective Reports of Precipitants to Relapse in Pathological Gambling. *Journal of Consulting and Clinical Psychology*, *72*(1), 72–80.

Hodgins, D., Peden, N., & Cassidy, E. (2005). The Association Between Comorbidity and Outcome in Pathological Gambling: A Prospective Follow-Up of Recent Quitters. *Journal of Gambling Studies*, *21*, 255–271.

Hodgins, D., Stea, J. & Grant, J. (2011). Gambling Disorders. *The Lancet*, *378* (e9-e10), 1874–1884.

Hodgins, D., Toneatto, T., Makarchuk, K., Skinner, W., & Vincent, S. (2007). Minimal Treatment Approaches for Concerned Significant Others of Problem Gamblers: A Randomized Controlled Trial. *Journal of Gambling Studies*, *23*(2), 215–230. doi: 10.1007/s10899-006-9052-2

Holdsworth, L., Haw, J., & Hing, N. (2012). The Temporal Sequencing of Problem Gambling and Comorbid Disorders. *International Journal of Mental Health and Addiction*, *10*(2), 197–209.

Holdsworth, L., & Tiyce, M. (2013). Untangling the Complex Needs of People Experiencing Gambling Problems and Homelessness. *International Journal of Mental Health and Addiction*, *11*(2), 186–198.

Holtgraves, T. (2009a). Gambling, Gambling Activities, and Problem Gambling. *Psychology of Addictive Behaviors*, *23*(2), 295.

Holtgraves, T. (2009b). Evaluating the Problem Gambling Severity Index. *Journal of Gambling Studies*, *25*(1), 105–120.

Hopley, A., Dempsey, K., & Nicki, R. (2011). Texas Hold'em Online Poker: A Further Examination. *International Journal of Mental Health and Addiction*, *10*(4), 563–572.

Horch, J. D., & Hodgins, D. C. (2015). Self-Stigma Coping and Treatment-Seeking in Problem Gambling. *International Gambling Studies, 15*(3), 470–488. http://dx.doi.org/10.1080/14459795.2015.1078392

Horváth, C., & Paap, R. (2012). The Effect of Recessions on Gambling Expenditures. *Journal of Gambling Studies, 28*(4), 703–717. https://www.ncbi.nlm.nih.gov/pmc/articles/PMC3501160/

HMRC [Her Majesty's Revenue & Customs]. (2013). Gambling Tax Reform 2014. Information note December 2013. HM Revenue & Customs in the UK.

Huang, G. H. (2011). Responsible Gambling Policies and Practices in Macao: A Critical Review. *Asian Journal of Gambling Issues and Public Health, 2*(1), 49–60. doi: 10.1186/BF03342125

Huberfeld, R., & Dannon, P. N. (2014). Pathological Gambling: Who Gains from Others' Losses? in E. Bijleveld, & H. Aarts, eds., *The Psychological Science of Money.* New York: Springer, 163–185.

Huizinga, J. (1938). *Homo Ludens: Essai sur la Fonction Sociale du Jeu.* Paris: Gallimard.

Humphreys, B. R., & Soebbing, B. P. (2014). Access to Legal Gambling and the Incidence of Crime: Evidence from Alberta. *Growth and Change, 45*(1), 98–120.

Humphreys, K., Wing, S., McCarty, D., Chappel, J., Gallant, L., Haberle, B., … & Laudet, A. (2004). Self-Help Organizations for Alcohol and Drug Problems: Toward Evidence-Based Practice and Policy. *Journal of Substance Abuse Treatment, 26*(3), 151–158.

Ibanez, A., Blanco, C., Donahue, E., Lesieur, H. R., Perez de Castro, I., Fernandez-Piqueras, J., et al. (2001). Psychiatric Comorbidity in Pathological Gamblers Seeking Treatment. *American Journal of Psychiatry, 158*(10), 1733–1735.

ICF-CNR (2014). Italian Population Survey on Alcohol and other Drugs—IPSAD® 2013–2014.

iGaming Business (2016). Italy Reveals Significant Online Gaming Growth in 2015. *iGambing Business*, February 1, 2016. http://www.igamingbusiness.com/news/italy-reveals-significant-online-gaming-growth-2015

Institut für Therapieforschung (IFT), & Bundesministerium für Gesundheit und soziale Sicherung (2011). *Epidemiological Survey on Substance Abuse in Germany 2009* (ESA). GESIS Data Archive, Cologne. doi: 10.4232/1.10772

Institute of Medicine (1988). *The Future of Public Health.* Washington, DC: National Academies Press. doi: https://doi.org/10.17226/1091

Jackson, A. C., Thomas, S. A., Thomason, N., & Ho, W. (2002). *Longitudinal Evaluation of the Effectiveness of Problem Gambling Counselling Services, Community Education Strategies and Information Products—Volume 3: Community Education Strategies and Information Products.* Melbourne, Australia: Victorian Department of Human Services.

Jacobs, D. F., Marston A. R., Singer, R. D., Widaman, K., Little, T. & Veizades, J. (1989). Children of Problem Gamblers. *Journal of Gambling Behavior, 5*(4), 261–268.

Jacques, C., & Ladouceur, R. (2006). A Prospective Study of the Impact of Opening a Casino on Gambling Behaviours: 2- and 4-Year Follow-Ups. *The Canadian Journal of Psychiatry, 51*(12), 764–773.

Jason, J., Taff, M., & Boglioli, L. (1990). Casino-Related Deaths in Atlantic City, New Jersey: 1982–1986. *Am. J. Forensic Med. Pathol. 11*, 112–123.

Jensen, C. (2017). Money Over Misery: Restrictive Gambling Legislation in an Era of Liberalization. *Journal of European Public Policy, 24*(1), 119–134. http://dx.doi.org/10.1080/13501763.2016.1146326

Jiménez-Murcia, S., Tremblay, J., Stinchfield, R. et al. (2016). The Involvement of a Concerned Significant Other in Gambling Disorder Treatment Outcome. *Journal of Gambling Studies*, First Online November, 17 doi: 10.1007/s10899-016-9657-z.

Johansson, A., Grant, J. E., Kim, S. W., Odlaug, B. L., & Götestam, K. G. (2009). Risk Factors for Problematic Gambling: A Critical Literature Review. *Journal of Gambling Studies*, 25(1), 67–92.

Johnson, L. T., & Ratcliffe, J. H. (2014). A Partial Test of the Impact of a Casino on Neighborhood Crime. *Security Journal*, 30(2), 437–453.

Kalischuk, R. G., Nowatzki, N., Cardwell, K., Klein, K., & Solowoniuk, J. (2006). Problem Gambling and its Impact on Families: A Literature Review. *International Gambling Studies*, 6(1), 31–60.

Karter, L. (2013). *Women and Problem Gambling: Therapeutic Insights Into Understanding Addiction and Treatment.* London: Routledge.

Kassinove, J. & Schare, M. (2001). Effects of the Near Miss and the Big Win on Persistence at Slot Machine Gambling. *Psychology of Addictive Behaviors*, 15(2), 155–158.

Kassinove, J. I., Tsytsarev, S. V., & Davidson, I. (1998). Russian Attitudes Toward Gambling. *Personality and Individual Differences*, 24(1), 41–46.

Kaufman, A., Nielsen, J. & Bowden-Jones, H. (2016). Barriers to Treatment for Female Problem Gamblers: A UK Perspective. *Journal of Gambling Studies*, First Online, December, 22, doi: 10.1007/s10899-016-9663-1.

Kavanagh, T. (2005). *Dice, Cards, Wheels. A Different History of French Culture.* Philadelphia: University of Pennsylvania Press.

Keen, B., Pickering, D., Wieczorek, M., & Blaszczynski, A. (2015). Problem Gambling and Family Violence in the Asian Context: A Review. *Asian Journal of Gambling Issues and Public Health*, 5(1), 1–16.

Kennedy, S. H., Welsh, B. R., Fulton, K., Soczynska, J. K., McIntyre, R. S., O'Donovan, C., … & Martin, N. (2010). Frequency and Correlates of Gambling Problems in Outpatients with Major Depressive Disorder and Bipolar Disorder. *The Canadian Journal of Psychiatry*, 55(9), 568–576.

Kessler, R. C., Hwang, I., LaBrie, R., Petukhova, M., Sampson, N. A., Winters, K. C., et al. (2008). DSM-IV Pathological Gambling in the National Comorbidity Survey Replication. *Psychological Medicine*, 38(9), 1351–1360.

Kim, J., Ahlgren, M. B., Byun, J. W., & Malek, K. (2016). Gambling Motivations and Superstitious Beliefs: A Cross-Cultural Study with Casino Customers. *International Gambling Studies*, 16(2), 296–315.

Kingma S. (2015). Paradoxes of Risk Management. Social Responsibility and Self-Exclusion in Dutch Casinos. *Culture and Organisation*, 21(1), 1–22.

Kingma, S. (2008). The Liberalization and (Re)Regulation of Dutch Gambling Markets: National Consequences of the Changing European Context. *Regulation & Governance*, 2(4), 445–458.

Kingma, S. (2004). Gambling and the Risk Society: The Liberalisation and Legitimation Crisis of Gambling in the Netherlands. *International Gambling Studies*, 4(1), 47–67.

Komoto, Y. (2014). Factors Associated with Suicide and Bankruptcy in Japanese Pathological Gamblers. *International Journal of Mental Health and Addiction*, 12(5), 600–606.

Koo, J., Rosentraub, M. S., & Horn, A. (2007). Rolling the Dice? Casinos, Tax Revenues, and the Social Costs of Gaming. *Journal of Urban Affairs, 29*(4), 367–381.

Korn, D. (2000). Expansion of Gambling in Canada: Implications for Social and Health Policy. *Canadian Medical Association Journal 163*(1), 61–64.

Korn, D., Gibbins, R., & Azmier, J. (2003). Framing Public Policy Towards a Public Health Paradigm for Gambling. *Journal of Gambling Studies, 19*(2), 235–256.

Korn, D., Hurson, T., & Reynolds, J. (2005). *Commercial Gambling Advertising: Possible Impact on Youth Knowledge, Attitudes, Beliefs and Behavioural Intentions.* Guelph: Ontario Problem Gambling Research Centre.

Korn, D., & Shaffer, H. (1999). Gambling and the Health of the Public: Adopting a Public Health Perspective. *Journal of Gambling Studies, 15*(4), 289–365. doi: 10.1023/A:1023005115932

KPMG Consulting (2002). Problem Gambling—ATM/EFTPOS Functions and Capabilities. Department of Family and Community Services. https://www.dss.gov.au/sites/default/files/documents/05_2012/problem_gambling.pdf.

Kuoppamäki, S. M., Kääriäinen, J., & Lind, K. (2014). Examining Gambling-Related Crime Reports in the National Finnish Police Register. *Journal of Gambling Studies, 30*(4), 967–983.

Kyngdon, A., & Dickerson, M. (1999). An Experimental Study of the Effect of Prior Alcohol Consumption on a Simulated Gambling Activity. *Addiction, 94*(5), 697–707. doi: 10.1046/j.1360-0443.1999.9456977.x

Ladd, G., & Petry, N. (2003). A Comparison of Pathological Gamblers With and Without Substance Abuse Treatment Histories. *Experimental and Clinical Psychopharmacology, 11*(3), 202–209.

Ladouceur, R., Blaszczynski, A., & Lalande, D. (2012). Pre-Commitment in Gambling: A Review of the Empirical Evidence. *International Gambling Studies, 12*(2), 215–230. http://dx.doi.org/10.1080/14459795.2012.658078

Ladouceur, R., Boutin, C., Doucet, C., Dumont, M., Provencher, M., Giroux, I., et al. (2004). Awareness Promotion About Excessive Gambling Among Video Lottery Retailers. *Journal of Gambling Studies, 20*(2), 181–185. doi: 10.1023/B:JOGS.0000022309.25027.25

Ladouceur, R., Jacques, C., Giroux, I., Ferland, F., & Leblond, J. (2000). Brief Communications Analysis of a Casino's Self-Exclusion Program. *Journal of Gambling Studies, 16*(4), 453–460. https://link.springer.com/article/10.1023/A:1009488308348

Ladouceur, R., Jacques, C., Sévigny, S., & Cantinotti, M. (2005). Impact of the Format, Arrangement, and Availability of Electronic Gaming Machines Outside Casinos on Gambling. *International Gambling Studies, 5*(2), 139–154. http://dx.doi.org/10.1080/14459790500303121

Ladouceur, R. & Mayrand, M. (1987). The Level of Involvement and the Timing of Betting in Roulette. *Journal of Psychology, 121*(2), 169–176. http://dx.doi.org/10.1080/00223980.1987.9712654

Ladouceur, R. & Sévigny, S. (2009). Electronic Gambling Machines: Influence of a Clock, a Cash Display, and a Precommitment on Gambling Time. *Journal of Gambling Issues, 23*, 31–41.

Ladouceur, R. & Sévigny, S. (2006). The Impact of Video Lottery Game Speed on Gamblers. *Journal of Gambling Issues, 17*. https://doi.org/10.4309/jgi.2006.17.12

Ladouceur, R., Sylvain, C., & Gosselin, P. (2007). Self-Exclusion Program: A Longitudinal Evaluation Study. *Journal of Gambling Studies*, *23*(1), 85–94. doi: 10.1007/s10899-006-9032-6

Laffey, D., Della Sala, V., & Laffey, K. (2016). Patriot Games: The Regulation of Online Gambling in the European Union. *Journal of European Public Policy*, *23*(10), 1425–1441.

Lähteenmaa, J. & Strand, T. (2008). *Pelin Jälkeen—Velkaa Vai Voittoja?* [*After the game—debts or gains*]. Helsinki: STAKES.

Lal, A., & Siahpush, M. (2008). The Effect of Smoke-Free Policies on Electronic Gaming Machine Expenditure in Victoria, Australia. *Journal of Epidemiological Community Health*, *62*(1), 11–15. http://dx.doi.org/10.1136/jech.2006.051557

Lam, D. (2014). *Chopsticks and Gambling*. New Jersey: Transaction Publishers.

Lambos, C., & Delfabbro, P. (2007). Numerical Reasoning Ability and Irrational Beliefs in Problem Gambling. *International Gambling Studies*, *7*(2), 157–171. http://dx.doi.org/10.1080/14459790701387428

Lang, K. & Omori, M. (2009). Can Demographic Variables Predict Lottery and Pari-Mutuel Losses? An Empirical Investigation. *Journal of Gambling Studies*, *25*(2): 171–183.

LaPlante, D., Gray, H., LaBrie, R., Kleschinsky, J., & Shaffer, H. (2012). Gaming Industry Employees' Responses to Responsible Gambling Training: A Public Health Imperative. *Journal of Gambling Studies*, *28*(2), 171–191. doi: 10.1007/s10899-011-9255-z

Lapuz, J., & Griffiths, M. (2010). The Role of Chips in Poker Gambling: An Empirical Pilot Study. *Gambling Research: Journal of the National Association for Gambling Studies* (Australia), *22*(1), 34–39.

Laursen, B., Plauborg, R., Ekholm, O., Larsen, C. V. L., & Juel, K. (2016). Problem Gambling Associated With Violent and Criminal Behaviour: A Danish Population-Based Survey and Register Study. *Journal of Gambling Studies*, **32**(1), 25–34.

Leblond, J. (2013). L'Irréalisme du Plan Budgétaire 2013–2014 pour Loto-Québec: Le Jeu Illegal [The unrealism of the Loto-Québec budget plan 2013–2014: Illegal gambling]

Ledermann, S. (1956). *Alcool, Alcoolisme, Alcoolisation. Données Scientifiques de Caractére Physiologique, Economique et Social*. Institute National d'Études Demographiques, Travaux et Documents, Cahier 29. Vol 1. Paris: Presses Universitaires de France.

Lee, H. (2002). *Psychology of Gambling*. Seoul: Hakjisa.

Leino, T., Torsheim, T., Blaszczynski, A., Griffiths, M., Mentzoni, R., Pallesen, S., & Molde, H. (2015). The Relationship Between Structural Game Characteristics and Gambling Behavior: A Population-Level Study. *Journal of Gambling Studies*, *31*(4), 1297–1315. doi: 10.1007/s10899-014-9477-y

Lemarié, L. (2012). *Three Essays on Pro- and Anti-Behavioural Messages in a Preventive Context*. Montréal: HEC.

Lepper, J. & Creigh-Tyte, S. W. (2013). The National Lottery, in L. Vaughan-Williams, D. S. Siegel eds., *The Oxford Handbook of the Economics of Gambling*. New York: Oxford University Press, 611–636.

Lesieur, H. (1994). Epidemiological Surveys of Pathological Gambling: Critique and Suggestions for Modification. *Journal of Gambling Studies*, *10*, 385–398.

Lesieur, H. R. (1990). Working With and Understanding Gamblers Anonymous, in T. J. Powell ed., *Working with self-help*. Silver Spring: NASW Press, 237–253.

Lesieur, H. R., Blume, S. B. (1987). The South Oaks Gambling Screen (SOGS): A New Instrument for the Identification of Pathological Gamblers. *American Journal of Psychiatry, 144*(9), 1184–1188.

Lhommeau, N., Alexandre, J. M., Mete, D., Fatseas, M., & Auriacombe, M. (2015). Characteristics of Gamblers Choosing Self-Exclusion from Casinos: A Prospective Study in a French Overseas Territory. *Drug & Alcohol Dependence, 156*, e127.

Li, E., Rockloff, M., Browne, M., & Donaldson, P. (2015). Jackpot Structural Features: Rollover Effect and Goal-Gradient Effect in EGM Gambling. *Journal of Gambling Studies, 32*(2), 707–720. doi: 10.1007/s10899-015-9557-7

Lind, K., Kääriäinen, J., & Kuoppamäki, S. M. (2015). From Problem Gambling to Crime? Findings from the Finnish National Police Information System. *Journal of Gambling Issues, 33*, 98–123.

Livingstone, C. (2007). Understanding the 'Community Benefit' of Electronic Gaming Machines: An Interim Analysis of Victorian EGM Community Benefit Statements. Melbourne: Monash University. http://www.parliament.vic.gov.au/images/stories/documents/council/Select_Committees/Gaming_Licensing/Submissions/GL10_Sup.pdf

Livingstone, C. (2005). Desire and Consumption of Danger: Electronic Gaming Machines and the Commodification of Interiority. *Addiction Research & Theory 13*(6), 523–534.

Livingstone, C., & Adams, P. J. (2016). Clear Principles are Needed for Integrity in Gambling Research. *Addiction, 111*(1), 5–10. doi: 10.1111/add.12913

Livingstone, C., & Adams, P. J. (2011). Harm Promotion: Observations on the Symbiosis Between Government and Private Industries in Australasia for the Development of Highly Accessible Gambling Markets. *Addiction, 106*(1), 3–8. doi: 10.1111/j.1360-0443.2010.03137.x. https://www.researchgate.net/profile/Angela_Rintoul/publication/266023628_What_is_the_evidence_for_harm_minimisation_measures_in_gambling_venues/links/542396a30cf238c6ea6e45c7.pdf

Livingstone, C., Woolley, R., Zazryn, T., Bakacs, L., & Shami, R. (2008). *The Relevance and Role of Gaming Machine Games and Game Features on the Play of Problem Gamblers.* Report for the Independent Gambling Authority, South Australia. Adelaide, SA: IGA.

Livingstone, C. & Woolley, R. (2007). Risky Business: A Few Provocations on the Regulation of Electronic Gambling Machines. *International Gambling Studies, 7*(3), 361–376.

Livingstone, D., Kipsaina, C., & Rintoul, A. (2012). Assessment of Poker Machine Expenditure and the Symbiosis Between Government and Private Industries in Australasia for the Development of Highly Accessible Gambling Markets. *Addiction, 106*, 3–8.

Livingstone, C., Rintoul, A., & Francis, L. (2014). What is the Evidence for Harm Minimization Measures in Gambling Venues. *Evidence Base, 2*, 1–24.

Loba, P., Stewart, S., Klein, R., & Blackburn, J. (2001). Manipulations of the Features of Standard Video Lottery Terminal (VLT) Games: Effects in Pathological and Non-Pathological Gamblers. *Journal of Gambling Studies, 17*(4), 297–320. doi: 10.1023/A:1013639729908

López Viets, V. L., & Miller, W. R. (1997). Treatment Approaches for Pathological Gamblers. *Clinical Psychology Review, 17*(7), 689–702. https://doi.org/10.1016/S0272-7358(97)00031-7

Lorains, F. K., Cowlishaw, S., & Thomas, S. A. (2011). Prevalence of Comorbid Disorders in Problem and Pathological Gambling: Systematic Review and Meta-Analysis of Population Surveys. *Addiction, 106*(3), 490–498.

Lorenz, V. C. & Yaffee, R. A. (1989). Pathological Gamblers and Their Spouses: Problems in Interaction. *Journal of Gambling Behavior, 5*(2): 113–126.

Lorenz, V. C., & Yaffee, R. A. (1986). Pathological Gambling: Psychosomatic, Emotional and Marital Difficulties as Reported by the Gambler. *Journal of Gambling Behavior, 2*(1), 40–49.

Lotteriinspektionen (2015). *Spelmarknadens Utveckling I Sverige Och Internationellt 2015* [Gambling market development in Sweden and internationally 2015]. http://www.lotteriinspektionen.se/Global/Broschyrer/Spelmarknaden%202015.pdf.

Lucar, C., Wiebe, J. & Philander, K. (2013). *Monetary Limits Tools for Internet Gamblers: A Review of Their Availability, Implementation and Effectiveness Online.* Final report prepared for the Ontario Problem Gambling Research Centre. http://www.responsiblegambling.org/docs/research-reports/monetary-limits-tools-for-internet-gamblers.pdf?sfvrsn=8

Ludwig, M., Kraus, L., Muller, S., Braun, B., & Buhringer, G. (2012). Has Gambling Changed After Major Amendments of Gambling Regulations in Germany? A Propensity Score Analysis. *Journal of Behavioral Addictions 1*(4), 151–161. doi: 10.1556/JBA.1.2012.4.2

Lund, I. (2011). Irrational Beliefs Revisited: Exploring the Role of Gambling Preferences in the Development of Misconceptions in Gamblers. *Addiction Research & Theory, 19*(1), 40–46. http://dx.doi.org/10.3109/16066359.2010.493979

Lund I. (2009). Gambling Behaviour and the Prevalence of Gambling Problems in Adult EGM Gamblers When Egms Are Banned. A Natural Experiment. *Journal of Gambling Studies, 25,* 215–225.

Lund, I. (2008). The Population Mean and the Proportion of Frequent Gamblers: Is the Theory of Total Consumption Valid for Gambling? *Journal of Gambling Studies, 24*(2), 247–256.

Lund, I. (2006). Gambling and Problem Gambling in Norway: What Part Does the Gambling Machine Play? *Addiction Research & Theory, 14*(5), 475–491.

Lund, I., & Nordlund, S. (2003). *Gambling Behaviour and Gambling Problems in Norway.* Oslo: Norwegian Institute for Alcohol and Drug Research, SIRUS.

McCleary, R., Chew, K. S., Merrill, V., & Napolitano, C. (2002). Does Legalized Gambling Elevate the Risk of Suicide? An Analysis Of US Counties and Metropolitan Areas. *Suicide and Life-Threatening Behavior, 32*(2), 209–221.

McComb, J. L., Lee, B. K., & Sprenkle, D. H. (2009). Conceptualizing and Treating Problem Gambling as a Family Issue. *Journal of Marital and Family Therapy, 35*(4), 415–431.

McGowan, R. (2001). *Government and the Transformation of the Gaming Industry.* Northampton: Edward Elgar.

McGrath, D., & Barrett, S. (2009). The Comorbidity of Tobacco Smoking and Gambling: A Review of the Literature. *Drug and Alcohol Review, 28*(6), 676–681.

McIntyre, R. S., McElroy, S. L., Konarski, J. Z., Soczynska, J. K., Wilkins, K., & Kennedy, S. H. (2007). Problem Gambling in Bipolar Disorder: Results from the Canadian Community Health Survey. *Journal of affective disorders, 102*(1), 27–34.

MacLaren, V., Ellery, M., & Knoll, T. (2015). Personality, Gambling Motives and Cognitive Distortions in Electronic Gambling Machine Players. *Personality and Individual Differences, 73*, 24–28.

McMillen, J., Marshall, D., Ahmed, E., & Wenzel, M. (2004a). 2003 Victorian Longitudinal Community Attitudes Survey. GRP Report no 6. Melbourne, Australia.

McMillen, J., Marshall, D., & Murphy, L. (2004b). *The Use of ATMs in ACT Gaming Venues: An Empirical Study.* Australian National University: Centre for Gambling Research.

McMillen, J., & Pitt, S. (2005). *Review of the ACT Government's Harm Minimisation Measures.* The Australian National University, Centre for Gambling Research.

McMullan, J. L., & Kervin, M. (2012). Selling Internet Gambling: Advertising, New Media and the Content of Poker Promotion. *International Journal of Mental Health and Addiction, 10*(5), 622–645. doi: 10.1007/s11469-011-9336-3

McMullan, J. L., & Miller, D. (2010). Advertising the "New Fun-Tier": Selling Casinos to Consumers. *International Journal of Mental Health and Addiction, 8*(1), 35–50. doi: 10.1007/s11469-009-9201-9

McMullan, J. L., & Miller, D. (2009). Wins, Winning and Winners: The Commercial Advertising of Lottery Gambling. *Journal of Gambling Studies, 25*(3), 273–295. doi: 10.1007/s10899-009-9120-5

McMullan, J. L., & Miller, D. (2008). All In! The Commercial Advertising of Offshore Gambling on Television. *Journal of Gambling Issues, 22*, 230–251. https://doi.org/10.4309/jgi.2008.22.6

McMullan, J. L., & Rege, A. (2010). Online Crime and Internet Gambling. *Journal of Gambling Issues, 24*(5), 54–85. doi: 10.4309/jgi.2010.24.5

Mangham, C., Carney, G., Burnett, S., & Williams, R. (2007). Socioeconomic Impacts of New Gaming Venues in Four British Columbia Lower Mainland Communities. Final Report. Prepared for Gaming Policy and Enforcement Branch, Ministry of Public Safety & Solicitor General, Government of British Columbia. Victoria, BC: Blue Thorn Research and Analysis Group.

Mao, L. (2013). *Sports Gambling as Consumption: An Econometric Analysis of Demand for Sports Lottery.* University of Florida, ProQuest Dissertations Publishing.

Mao, L., Zhang, J., Connaughton, D., & Holland, S. (2015). An Examination of the Impact of Socio-Demographic Factors on the Demand for Sports Lotteries in China. *Asia Pacific Journal of Sport and Social Science, 4*(1), 34–52.

Marionneau, V., & Järvinen-Tassopoulos, J. (2017). Consumer Protection in Licensed Online Gambling Markets in France: The Role of Responsible Gambling Tools. *Addiction Research & Theory*, 1–8. http://dx.doi.org/10.1080/16066359.2017.1314464

Marionneau, V. & Nikkinen, J. (2017). Market Cannibalization Within and Between Gambling Industries: A Systematic Review. *Journal of Gambling Issues, 37*.

Markham, F. & Young, M. (2015). "Big Gambling": The Rise of the Global Industry State Gambling Complex. *Addiction Research and Theory, 23*(1), 1–4.

Markham, F. & Young, M. (2014). Who Wins from 'Big Gambling' in Australia? *The Conversation*, March 5, 2014. https://theconversation.com/who-wins-from-big-gambling-in-australia-22930

Markham, F., Young, M., & Doran, B. (2016). The Relationship Between Player Losses and Gambling-Related Harm: Evidence from Nationally Representative Cross-Sectional Surveys in Four Countries. *Addiction, 111*(2), 320–330.

Markham, F., Young, M., & Doran, B. (2014). Gambling Expenditure Predicts Harm: Evidence from a Venue-Level Study. *Addiction, 109*(9), 1509–1516.

Markham, F., Young, M., & Doran, B. (2012). The Relationship Between Alcohol Consumption, Gambling Behaviour and Problem Gambling During a Single Visit to a Gambling Venue. *Drug and Alcohol Review, 31*(6), 770–777. doi: 10.1111/j.1465-3362.2012.00430.x

Marshall, D. (2009). Gambling and Organized Crime: A Review of the Literature. *Journal of Gambling Issues, 23,* 111–155.

Marshall, D. (2005). The Gambling Environment and Gambling Behaviour: Evidence from Richmond-Tweed, Australia. *International Gambling Studies, 5*(1), 63–83.

Marshall, D. C., & Baker, R. G. (2002). The Evolving Market Structures of Gambling: Case Studies Modelling the Socioeconomic Assignment Of Gaming Machines in Melbourne and Sydney, Australia. *Journal of Gambling Studies, 18*(3), 273–291.

Marshall K., & Wynne, H. (2004). Against the Odds: A Profile of At-Risk and Problem Gamblers. *Canadian Social Trends* **2004,** 25–9.

Martins, S., Ghandour, L., Lee, G., & Storr, C. (2010). Sociodemographic and Substance Use Correlates of Gambling Behavior in the Canadian General Population. *Journal of Addictive Diseases, 29*(3), 338–351.

Martins S., Storr C., Lee G., & Ialongo, N. (2013). Environmental Influences Associated With Gambling in Young Adulthood. *Journal of Urban Health, 90*(1), 130–140.

Mathews, M., & Volberg, R. (2013). Impact of Problem Gambling on Financial, Emotional and Social Well-Being of Singaporean Families. *International Gambling Studies, 13*(1), 127–140.

Matilainen, R. (2010). A Question of Money? The Founding of Two Finnish Gambling Monopolies, in S. Kingma, ed., *Global gambling: Cultural Perspectives On Gambling Organisation.* New York: Routledge.

Matuszewski, E. (2014). Daily Fantasy Sites Buy Sponsorship to Build on $1 Billion Fees. *Bloomberg,* December 18, 2014. Online. http://www.bloomberg.com/news/articles/2014-12-18/daily-fantasy-sites-buy-sponsorships-to-build-on-1-billion-fees

Medeiros, G., Grant, J., & Tavares, H. (2016). Gambling Disorder Due to Brazilian Animal Game (Jogo de Bicho): Gambling Behaviour and Psychopathology. *Journal of Gambling Studies, 32*(1), 231–241.

Meier, P. (2010). Polarized Drinking Patterns and Alcohol Deregulation. *Nordic Studies on Alcohol and Drugs, 27*(5), 383–408.

Mentzoni, R., Laberg, J., Brunborg, G., Molde, H., & Pallesen, S. (2012). Tempo in Electronic Gaming Machines Affects Behavior Among At-Risk Gamblers. *Journal of Behavioral Addictions, 1*(3), 135–139. https://doi.org/10.1556/JBA.1.2012.004

Meyer, G., & Bachmann, M. (2011). *Spielsucht. Ursachen, Therapie und Prävention von glücksspielbezogenem Suchtverhalten* (3rd edn). Berlin: Springer.

Meyer, G., Häfeli, J., Mörsen, C., & Fiebig, M. (2010). Die Einschätzung des Gefährdungspotenzials von Glücksspielen. *Sucht, 56*(6), 405–414. https://doi.org/10.1024/0939-5911/a000057

Meyer, G., Hayer, T., & Griffiths, M. eds. (2009). *Problem Gambling in Europe.* New York: Springer.

Miller, J. D., MacKillop, J., Fortune, E. E., Maples, J., Lance, C. E., Campbell, W. K., et al. (2013). Personality Correlates of Pathological Gambling Derived from Big Three and Big Five Personality Models. *Psychiatry Research, 206*(1), 50–55.

Moghaddam, J. F., Yoon, G., Dickerson, D. L., Kim, S. W., & Westermeyer, J. (2015). Suicidal Ideation and Suicide Attempts in Five Groups with Different Severities of Gambling: Findings from the National Epidemiologic Survey on Alcohol and Related Conditions. *The American Journal on Addictions*, 24(4), 292–298.

Monaghan, S. (2008). Review of Pop-Up Messages on Electronic Gaming Machines as a Proposed Responsible Gambling Strategy. *International Journal of Mental Health and Addiction*, 6(2), 214–222. doi: 10.1007/s11469-007-9133-1

Monaghan, S. & Blaszczynski, A. (2010a). Electronic Gaming Machine Warning Messages: Information Versus Self-Evaluation. *Journal of Psychology: Interdisciplinary and Applied*, 144(1), 83–96.

Monaghan, S. & Blaszczynski, A. (2010b). Impact of Mode Display and Message Content of Responsible Gambling Signs for Electronic Gaming Machines on Regular Gamblers. *Journal of Gambling Studies*, 26(1), 67–88.

Monaghan, S. & Blaszczynski, A. (2007). Recall of Electronic Gaming Machine Signs: A Static Versus a Dynamic Mode of Presentation. *Journal of Gambling Issues*, 20, 253–267. https://doi.org/10.4309/jgi.2007.20.8

Monaghan, S., Derevensky, J., & Sklar, A. (2008). Impact of Gambling Advertisements and Marketing on Children and Adolescents: Policy Recommendations to Minimise Harm. *Journal of Gambling Issues*, 22, 252–274. https://doi.org/10.4309/jgi.2008.22.7

Moore, S., Thomas, A., Kyrios, M., Bates, G., & Meredyth, D. (2011). Gambling Accessibility: A Scale to Measure Gambler Preference. *Journal of Gambling Studies*, 27(1), 129–143.

Morasco, B., Pietrzak, R., Blanco, C, Grant, B., Hasin, D., & Petry, N. (2006). Health Problems and Medical Utilization Associated with Gambling Disorders: Results from the National Epidemiological Survey on Alcohol and Related Conditions. *Psychosomatic Medicine*, 68(6), 976–984.

National Research Council (1999). *Pathological Gambling: A Critical Review*. Washington, DC: The National Academies Press. doi:https://doi.org/10.17226/6329.

Nelson, S., LaPlante, D., Peller, A., Schumann, A., LaBrie, R., Shaffer, H. (2008). Real Limits in the Virtual World: Self-Limiting Behavior of Internet Gamblers. *Journal of Gambling Studies*, 24(4), 463–477. doi: 10.1007/s10899-008-9106-8

Neurisse, A. (1991). *Les Jeux d'Argent et de Hasard*. Paris: Éditions Hermé.

New South Wales. Department of Gaming and Racing & AC Nielsen Company (Australia) (2003). Evaluation of the Impact of the Three Hour Shutdown of Gaming Machines: Final Report. AC Nielsen, Sydney, NSW.

Newman, S. C. (2007). The Association Between Pathological Gambling and Attempted Suicide: Findings from a National Survey in Canada. *Canadian Journal of Psychiatry*, 52(9), 605.

Nibert, D. (2000). *Hitting the Lottery Jackpot: State Governments and the Taxing of Dreams*. New York: Monthly Review Press.

Norsk Tipping (2016). https://www.norsk-tipping.no/selskapet/overskudd-og-sponsorater/overskudd

Norström, T., & Ramstedt, M. (2005). Mortality and Population Drinking: A Review of the Literature. *Drug and Alcohol Review*, 24(6), 537–547.

Noseworthy, T., & Finlay, K. (2009). A Comparison of Ambient Casino Sound and Music: Effects on Dissociation and on Perceptions of Elapsed Time While Playing Slot Machines. *Journal of Gambling Studies*, 25(3), 331–342.

Nova Scotia Gaming Corporation (2005). VLT Time Change: Findings Report.

Odlaug, B. L., Schreiber, L. R., & Grant, J. E. (2012). Personality Disorders and Dimensions in Pathological Gambling. *Journal of Personality Disorders*, *26*(3), 381–392.

Oei, T. P. S., & Raylu, N. (2004). Familial Influence on Offspring Gambling: A Cognitive Mechanism for Transmission of Gambling Behavior in Families. *Psychological Medicine*, *34*(7), 1279–1288.

Ofcom (2013). Trends in Advertising Activity—Gambling. London: Independent Regulator and Competition Authority for the UK Communications Industries http://stakeholders.ofcom.org.uk/binaries/research/tv-research/Trends_in_Ad_Activity_Gambling.pdf

Omnifacts Bristol Research (2007). *Nova Scotia Player Card Research Project. Stage III Research Report*. Report prepared for Nova Scotia Gaming Corporation.

Omnifacts Bristol Research (2005). *Nova Scotia Player Card Research Project: Stage I Research Project*. Report prepared for Nova Scotia Gaming Corporation.

Orford, J. (2017). How Does the Common Core to the Harm Experienced by Affected Family Members Vary by Relationship, Social and Cultural Factors? *Drugs: Education, Prevention and Policy*, *24*(1), 9–16.

Orford, J. (2012). Gambling in Britain: An Application of Erosion Theory. *Addiction*, *107*(12), 2082–2086. doi: 10.1111/j.1360-0443.2012.03821.x

Orford, J. (2010). *An Unsafe Bet? The Dangerous Rise of Gambling and the Debate We Should Be Having*. New Jersey: John Wiley & Sons.

Orford, J. (2008). Asking the Right Questions in the Right Way: The Need for a Shift in Research on Psychological Treatments for Addiction. *Addiction*, *103*(6), doi: 875–885. 10.1111/j.1360-0443.2007.02092.x

Orford, J., Sproston, K., & Erens, B. (2003a). SOGS and DSM-IV in the British Gambling Prevalence Survey: Reliability and Factor Structure. *International Gambling Studies*, *3*(1), 53–65.

Orford, J., Sproston, K., Erens, B., White, C., & Mitchell, L. (2003b) *Gambling and Problem Gambling in Britain*. Hove and New York: Brunner-Routledge

Orford, J., Templeton, L., Velleman, R., & Copello, A. (2005). Family Members of Relatives with Alcohol, Drug and Gambling Problems: A Set of Standardized Questionnaires for Assessing Stress, Coping and Strain. *Addiction*, *100*(11), 1611–1624.

Orford, J., Wardle, H., & Griffiths, M. (2013). What Proportion of Gambling is Problem Gambling? Estimates from the 2010 British Gambling Prevalence Survey. *International Gambling Studies*, *13*(1), 4–18.

Paldam, M. (2008). The Political Economy of Regulating Gambling: Illustrated with the Danish case, in M. Viren ed., *Gaming in the New Market Environment*. London: Palgrave Macmillan, 184–208.

Paloheimo, E. (2010). Verkkorahapelien Vetovoimatekijät [Attractions of Internet Gambling] *Pelitutkimuksen vuosikirja* 2010, 33–41. http://www.pelitutkimus.fi/vuosikirja2010/ptvk2010-04.pdf

Panichi, J. (2013). The Lobby Group that Got Much More Bang for its Buck. http://insidestory.org.au/the-lobby-group-that-got-much-more-bang-for-its-buck

Paoli, L. ed., (2014). *The Oxford Handbook of Organized Crime*. Oxford: Oxford University Press.

Papineau, E., Lemétayer, F., Barry, A., & Biron, J. (2015). Lottery Marketing in Québec and Social Deprivation: Excessive Exposure, Insufficient Protection? *International Gambling Studies, 15*(1), 88–107.

Parhami, I., Mojtabai, R., Rosenthal, R. J., Afifi, T. O., & Fong, T. W. (2014). Gambling and the Onset of Comorbid Mental Disorders: A Longitudinal Study Evaluating Severity and Specific Symptoms. *Journal of Psychiatric Practice, 20*(3), 207–219.

Park, S., Cho, M. J., Jeon, H. J., Lee, H. W., Bae, J. N., Park, J. I., Sohn, J. H., Lee, Y. R., Lee, J. Y., & Hong, J. P. (2010). Prevalence, Clinical Correlations, Comorbidities, and Suicidal Tendencies in Pathological Korean Gamblers: Results from the Korean Epidemiologic Catchment Area Study. *Social Psychiatry and Psychiatric Epidemiology, 45*(6), 621–629.

Parke, A., & Griffiths, M. (2004). Aggressive Behaviour in Slot Machine Gamblers: A Preliminary Observational Study. *Psychological Reports, 95*(1), 109–114.

Parke, A., Harris, A., Goddard, P., & Parke, J. (2014). *The Role of Stake Size in Loss of Control in Within-Session Gambling. Impact of Stake Size on Reflection Impulsivity, Response Inhibition and Arousal when Gambling on a Simulated Virtual Roulette Gambling Task: Implications for Gambling Related Harm.* Technical Report. Responsible Gambling Trust. http://eprints.lincoln.ac.uk/16410/1/Stake%20Size%20Report.pdf

Parke, J., & Parke, A. (2013). Does Size Really Matter? A Review of the Role of Stake and Prize Levels in Relation to Gambling-Related Harm. *Journal of Gambling Business and Economics, 7*(3), 77–110.

Parke, J., & Griffiths, M. (2006). The Psychology of the Fruit Machine: The Role of Structural Characteristics (Revisited). *International Journal of Mental Health and Addiction, 4*(2), 151–179. doi: 10.1007/s11469-006-9014-z

Parvulesco, C. (2008). *Casino—Plaisir du Jeu*. Boulogne-Billancourt: Du May.

Patford, J. (2009). For Worse, For Poorer and Ill Health: How Women Experience, Understand and Respond to a Partner's Gambling Problems. *International Journal of Mental Health and Addictions, 7*(1), 177–189.

Patford, J. (2007). For Poorer: How Men Experience, Understand and Respond to Problematic Aspects of a Partner's Gambling. *Gambling Research, 19*(1 and 2), 7–20.

Pearce, J., Mason, K., Hiscock, R. & Day, P. (2008). A National Study of Neighbourhood Access to Gambling Opportunities and Individual Gambling Behaviour. *Journal of Epidemiology and Community Health, 62*(10), 862–868.

Petry, N. M. (2005). *Pathological Gambling: Etiology, Comorbidity, and Treatment*. American Psychological Association.

Petry, N. M. (2003). A Comparison of Treatment-Seeking Pathological Gamblers Based on Preferred Gambling Activity. *Addiction, 98*(5), 645–655. doi: 10.1046/j.1360-0443.2003.00336.x

Petry, N. M., Blanco, C., Auriacombe, M., Borges, G., Bucholz, K., Crowley, T. J., … O'Brien, C. (2014). An Overview of and Rationale for Changes Proposed for Pathological Gambling in DSM-5. *Journal of Gambling Studies, 30*(2), 493–502.

Petry, N., & Oncken, C. (2002). Cigarette Smoking is Associated with Increased Severity of Gambling Problems in Treatment-Seeking Gamblers. *Addiction, 97*(6), 745–753. doi: 10.1046/j.1360-0443.2002.00163.x

Petry, N. M., Stinson, F. S. and **Grant, B. F.** (2005). Comorbidity of DSM–IV Pathological Gambling and Other Psychiatric Disorders: Results from the National Epidemiologic Survey on Alcohol and Related Conditions. *Journal of Clinical Psychiatry*, *66*, 564–574.

Petry, N., Weinstock, J., Ledgerwood, D. M., & **Morasco, B.** (2008). A Randomized Trial of Brief Interventions for Problem and Pathological Gamblers. *J Consult Clin Psychol*. *76*(2), 318–328. doi: 10.1037/0022-006X.76.2.318

Philander, K., & **Mackay, T.** (2014). Online Gambling Participation and Problem Gambling Severity: Is there a Causal Relationship? *International Gambling Studies*, *14*(2), 214–227.

Phillips, D. P., Welty, W. R., & **Smith, M. M.** (1997). Elevated Suicide Levels Associated with Legalized Gambling. *Suicide and Life-threatening Behavior*, *27*(4), 373–378.

Piedallu, J. (2014). Le Jeu Sous Contrôle. Analyse Sociologique des Formes de Régulations a l'oeuvre Dans la Pratique Contemporaine du Poker en France. Ph.D. Thesis. Paris: Université Paris Descartes.

Pietrzak, R. H., & **Petry, N. M.** (2005). Antisocial Personality Disorder is Associated with Increased Severity of Gambling, Medical, Drug and Psychiatric Problems Among Treatment-Seeking Pathological Gamblers. *Addiction*, *100*(8), 1183–1193.

Pirog-Good, M., & **Mikesell, J. L.** (1995). Longitudinal Evidence of the Changing Socio-Economic Profile of a State Lottery Market. *Policy Studies Journal*, *23*(3), 451–465.

Planzer, S. (2014). *Empirical Views on European Gambling Law and Addiction. Studies in European Economic Law and Regulation*. Cham, Switzerland: Springer.

Planzer, S., Gray, H. M., & **Shaffer, H. J.** (2014). Associations Between National Gambling Policies and Disordered Gambling Prevalence Rates Within Europe. *International Journal of Law and Psychiatry*, *37*(2), 217–229. https://doi.org/10.1016/j.ijlp.2013.11.002

Planzer, S. & **Wardle, H.** (2011). *The Comparative Effectiveness of Regulatory Approaches and the Impact of Advertising on Propensity for Problem Gambling*. London: Responsible Gambling Fund.

Polders, B. (1997). Gambling in Europe—Unity in Diversity, in W. R. Eadington & J. A. Cornelius, eds., *Gambling: Public Policies and the Social Sciences*. Reno: Institute for the Study of Gambling and Commercial Gaming, University of Nevada, 65–100.

Pontell, H., Fang, Q., & **Geis, G.** (2014). Economic Crime and Casinos: China's Wager on Macau. *Asian Journal of Criminology*, *9*(1), 1–13.

Potenza, M., Fiellin, D., Heninger, G., Rounsaville, B. M & **Mazure, C.** (2002). Gambling: An Addictive Behavior with Health and Primary Care Implications. *Journal of General Internal Medicine*, *17*(9), 721–732.

Potenza, M., Steinberg, M., McLaughlin, S., Wu, R., Rounsaville, B., & **O'Malley, S.** (2001). Gender-Related Differences in the Characteristics of Problem Gamblers Using a Gambling Helpline. *American Journal of Psychiatry*, *158*(9), 1500–1505.

Price D., & **Novak E.** (1999). The Tax Incidence of Three Texas Lottery Games: Regressivity, Race, and Education. *National Tax Journal*, *52*, 741–751.

Pryor, F. (1976). The Friedman–Savage Utility Function in Cross-Cultural Perspective. *Journal of Political Economy*, *84*(4, part 1), 821–834.

Qi, S., Ding, C., Song, Y., & **Yang, D.** (2011). Neural Correlates of Near-Misses Effect in Gambling. *Neuroscience Letters*, *493*(3), 80–85. https://doi.org/10.1016/j.neulet.2011.01.059

Queensland Government Statistician's Office (2016). Australian Gambling Statistics 1989–90 to 2014–15, 32nd edition. http://www.qgso.qld.gov.au/products/reports/aus-gambling-stats/aus-gambling-stats-32nd-edn.pdf

Queensland Government Treasury 2007. Australian Gambling Statistics: 1980–81 to 2005–06, 24th edition.

Quigley, L., Yakovenko, I., Hodgins, D. C., Dobson, K. S., el-Guebaly, N., Casey, D. M., & Schopflocher, D. P. (2015). Comorbid Problem Gambling and Major Depression in a Community Sample. *Journal of Gambling Studies, 31*(4), 1135–1152.

Rahman, A. S., Pilver, C. E., Desai, R. A., Steinberg, M. A., Rugle, L., Krishnan-Sarin, S., & Potenza, M. N. (2012). The Relationship Between Age of Gambling Onset and Adolescent Problematic Gambling Severity. *Journal of Psychiatric Research, 46*(5), 675–683.

Raisamo, S. U., Mäkelä, P., Salonen, A. H., & Lintonen, T. P. (2015a). The Extent and Distribution of Gambling Harm in Finland as Assessed by the Problem Gambling Severity Index. *The European Journal of Public Health, 25*(4), 716–722.

Raisamo, S., Warpenius, K. & Rimpelä, A. (2015b). Changes in Minors' Gambling on Slot Machines in Finland After the Raising of the Minimum Legal Gambling Age from 15 to 18 years: A Repeated Cross-Sectional Study. *Nordic Studies on Alcohol and Drugs, 32*(4), 579–590.

Rand, K. R., & Light, S. A. (2006). *Indian Gaming Law and Policy*. Durham, NC: Carolina Academic Press.

Raninen, J., Leifman, H., & Ramstedt, M. (2013). Who is Not Drinking Less in Sweden? An Analysis of the Decline in Consumption for the Period 2004–2011. *Alcohol and Alcoholism, 48*(5), 592–597.

Raninen J., Livingston, M., & Leifman, H. (2014). Declining Trends in Alcohol Consumption Among Swedish Youth—Does the Theory of Collectivity of Drinking Cultures Apply? *Alcohol and Alcoholism, 49*(6), 681–6.

Raylu, N., & Oei, T. (2002). Pathological Gambling: A Comprehensive Review. *Clinical Psychology Review, 22*(7), 1009–1061.

Reece, W. S. (2010). Casinos, Hotels, and Crime. *Contemporary Economic Policy, 28*(2), 145–161.

Rehm, J., Kehoe, T., Stinson, F., Grant, B., & Gmel, G. (2010). Statistical Modeling of Volume of Alcohol Exposure for Epidemiological Studies of Population Health: The US Example. *Population Health Metrics, 8*(1), 3.

Reith, G. (2006). The Pursuit of Chance, in James F. Cosgrave, ed., *The Sociology of Risk and Gambling Reader*. New York: Routledge, 125–142.

Reith, G. (1999). *The Age of Chance*. Oxford: Routledge.

Responsible Gambling Council (2015). *Canadian Gambling Digest 2013–2014. Canadian Partnership for Responsible Gambling*. http://www.responsiblegambling.org/docs/default-source/default-document-library/cprg_canadian-gambling-digest_2013-14.pdf?sfvrsn=2

Responsible Gambling Council (2008). *From Enforcement to Assistance: Evolving Best Practices in Self-Exclusion*. RGC Centre for the Advancement of Best Practices. http://www.responsiblegambling.org/docs/default-source/research-reports/

from-enforcement-to-assistance-evolving-best-practices-in-self-exclusion. pdf?sfvrsn=10

Responsible Gambling Council (2006). *Electronic Gaming Machines and Problem Gambling*. http://www.responsiblegambling.org/docs/research-reports/electronic-gaming-machines-and-problem-gambling.pdf?sfvrsn=10

Reynolds, B. (2006). A Review of Delay-Discounting Research with Humans: Relations to Drug Use and Gambling. *Behavioural Pharmacology, 17*(8), 651–667.

Robitaille, É., & Herjean, P. (2008). An Analysis of the Accessibility of Video Lottery Terminals: The Case of Montréal. *International Journal of Health Geographics, 7*(1), 2.

Rintoul, A. C., Deblaquiere, J., Thomas, A. (2017). Responsible gambling codes of conduct: lack of harm minimisation intervention in the context of venue self-regulation, *Addiction Research & Theory, 25*(6), 451–461. doi: 10.1080/16066359.2017.1314465

Rintoul, A. C., Livingstone, C., Mellor, A. P., Jolley, D. (2013). Modelling vulnerability to gambling related harm: How disadvantage predicts gambling losses. *Addiction Research & Theory, 21*(4), 329–338. doi: 10.3109/16066359.2012.727507

Rockloff, M., Donaldson, P., & Browne, M. (2015). Jackpot Expiry: An Experimental Investigation of a New EGM Player-Protection Feature. *Journal of Gambling Studies, 31*(3), 1505–1514. doi: 10.1007/s10899-014-9472-3

Rockloff, M., Greer, N., & Fay, C. (2011). The Social Contagion of Gambling: How Venue Size Contributes to Player Losses. *Journal of Gambling Studies, 27*(3), 487–497. doi: 10.1007/s10899-010-9220-2

Rockloff, M., & Hing, N. (2013). The Impact of Jackpots on EGM Gambling Behaviour: A Review. *Journal of Gambling Studies, 29*(4), 775–790.

Rodda, S., & Cowie, M. (2005). *Evaluation of Electronic Gaming Machine Harm Minimisation in Victoria*. Report prepared for the Victorian Department of Justice, Melbourne, Caraniche Pty. Ltd.

Rodda, S. N., Hing, N., & Lubman, D. I. (2014). Improved Outcomes Following Contact with a Gambling Helpline: The Impact of Gender on Barriers and Facilitators. *International Gambling Studies, 14*(2), 318–329. http://dx.doi.org/10.1080/14459795.2014.921721

Roerecke, M., & Rehm, J. (2014). Alcohol Consumption, Drinking Patterns, and Ischemic Heart Disease: A Narrative Review of Meta-Analyses and a Systematic Review and Meta-Analysis of the Impact of Heavy Drinking Occasions on Risk for Moderate Drinkers. *BMC Medicine, 12*(1), 182.

Rogers, P. (1998). The Cognitive Psychology of Lottery Gamblings. A Theoretical Review. *Journal of Gambling Studies, 14*(2), 111–134.

Rogers, P., & Webley, P. (2001). "It Could Be Us!": Cognitive and Social Psychological Factors in UK National Lottery Play. *Applied Psychology, 50*(1), 181–199.

Rolando, S. & Scavarda, A. (2016). *Gambling Policy in European Welfare Regimes. A European Research Project on the Profitability of Gambling. Italian Report*. Publications of the Faculty of Social Sciences, 30/2016. Helsinki: Unigrafia.

Room, R. & Cisneros Örnberg, J. (2014). The Governance of Addictions at the International Level, in P. Anderson et al. eds., *Reframing Addictions: Policies, Processes and Pressures*. Barcelona: ALICE RAP Project, 46–58.

Room, R., Turner, N., & Ialomiteanu, A. (1999). Community Effects of the Opening of the Niagara Casino. *Addiction, 94*(10), 1449–1466.

Rose, G., & Day, S. (1990). The Population Mean Predicts the Number of Deviant Individuals. *BMJ, 301*(6759), 1031–1034.

Rose, I. N. (1991). The Rise and Fall of the Third Wave: Gambling Will be Outlawed in Forty Years, in W. R. Eadington, & J. A. Cornelius eds., *Gambling and Public Policy: International Perspectives.* Reno: Institute for the Study of Gambling and Commercial Gaming, University of Nevada, 65–86.

Rosecrance, John (1985). Compulsive Gambling and the Medicalization of Deviance. *Social Problems, 32,* 275–284.

Rosenthal, F. (1975). *Gambling in Islam.* Leiden: E. J. Brill.

Rossow, I., & Clausen, T. (2013). The Collectivity of Drinking Cultures: Is the Theory Applicable to African Settings? *Addiction, 108*(9), 1612–1617.

Rossow, I., & Hansen, M. (2016). Gambling and Gambling Policy in Norway—An Exceptional Case. *Addiction, 111*(4), 593–598. doi: 10.1111/add.13172

Rossow, I., & Molde, H. (2006). Chasing the Criteria: Comparing SOGS-RA and the Lie/ Bet Screen to Assess Prevalence of Problem Gambling and "At-Risk"Gambling Among Adolescents. *Journal of Gambling Issues, 18,* 57–71.

Rossow, I., & Norström, T. (2013). The Use of Epidemiology in Alcohol Research. *Addiction, 108*(1), 20–25.

Rychtarik, R. G., & McGillicuddy, N. B. (2006). Preliminary Evaluation of a Coping Skills Training Program for Those with a Pathological-Gambling Partner. *Journal of Gambling Studies, 22*(2), 165–178. doi: 10.1007/s10899-006-9008-6

Sabbagh, J. J. (2013). *Drunk Gamblers: The Impact of Legalized Gambling on Alcohol Consumption.* Doctoral dissertation, Universidad de San Andrés.

St-Pierre, R., Walker, D., Derevensky, J., & Gupta, R. (2014). How Availability and Accessibility of Gambling Venues Influence Problem Gambling: A Review of the Literature. *Gaming Law Review and Economics, 18*(2), 150–172.

Sallaz, J. (2010). Gambling with Development. Comparing Casino Legalization in South Africa with Indian Gambling in California, in S. Kingma, ed., *Global Gambling: Cultural Perspectives on Gambling Organisation.* New York: Routledge, 64–88.

Salonen, A., Castrén, S., Alho, H., & Lahti, T. (2014). Concerned Significant Others of People with Gambling Problems in Finland: A Cross-Sectional Population Study. *BMC Public Health, 14*(1), 398–416.

Salonen, A., & Raisamo, S. (2015). *Suomalaisten rahapelaaminen 2015- Rahapelaaminen, rahapeliongelmat ja rahapelaamiseen liittyvät asenteet ja mielipiteet 15–74 -vuotiailla.* Raportti: 2015_016. [Gambling in Finland. Gambling, gambling problems and attitudes and opinions among the 15–74 year- old population] http://www.julkari.fi/bitstream/handle/10024/129595/URN_ISBN_ 978-952-302-559-2.pdf?sequence=1

Sandberg, H., Gidlöf, K. & Holmberg, N. 2011. Children's Exposure to and Perceptions of Online Advertising. *International Journal of Communication, 5,* 21–50.

Santangelo, G., Barone, P. Trojano, L., & Vitale, C. (2013). Pathological Gambling in Parkinson's Disease. A Comprehensive Review. *Parkinsonism & Related Disorders, 19*(7), 645–653. doi.org/10.1016/j.parkreldis.2013.02.007

Sassen, M., Kraus, L., & Bühringer, G. (2011a). Differences in Pathological Gambling Prevalence Estimates: Facts or Artefacts? *International Journal of Methods in Psychiatric Research, 20*(4), e83–e99.

Sassen, M., Kraus, L., Bühringer, G., Pabst, A., Piontek, D., & Taqi, Z. (2011b). Gambling Among Adults in Germany: Prevalence, Disorder and Risk Factors. SUCHT-Zeitschrift für Wissenschaft und Praxis/*Journal of Addiction Research and Practice*, *57*(4), 249–257.

Savage, A. (2014). Melbourne's Crown Casino has its License Extended to 2050. ABC News (Australian Broadcasting Corporation) August 22, 2014.

Schaap, J. (2010). The Growth of the Native American Gaming Industry: What has the Past Provided, and What Does the Future Hold? *The American Indian Quarterly*, *34*(3), 365–389. doi: 10.1353/aiq.0.0125

Schellinck, T., & Schrans, T. (2007). *VLT Player Tracking System*. Focal Research: Nova Scotia.

Schellinck, T., & Schrans, T. (2002). *Atlantic Lottery Corporation Video Lottery Responsible Gaming Feature Research: Final report*. Focal Research Consultants Ltd.

Schellinck, T., & Schrans, T. (2010). *Evaluating the Impact of the "My-Play" System in Nova Scotia*. Nova Scotia Gaming Foundation.

Schissel, B. (2001). Betting Against Youth: The Effects of Socioeconomic Marginality on Gambling among Young People. *Youth & Society*, *32*(4), 473–491.

Schluter, P., Bellringer, M., & Abbott, M. (2007). Maternal Gambling Associated with Families' Food, Shelter, and Safety Needs: Findings from the Pacific Island Families Study. *Journal of Gambling Issues*, *19*, 87–90.

Schneider, F. (2013). Money Laundering & Online Poker: How Relevant?. *Gaming Law Review and Economics*, *17*(10), 714–727.

Schottler Consulting (2010). *Major Findings and Implications: Player Tracking and Pre-Commitment Trial: A Program and Outcome Evaluation of the PlaySmart Precommitment System*. http://www.treasury.sa.gov.au/__data/assets/pdf_file/0016/2158/PlaySmart.pdf

Schottler Consulting (2009). *Major findings of a trial of a card-based gaming product at the Redcliffe RSL*. http://www.greo.ca/Modules/EvidenceCentre/Details/major-findings-trial-card-based-gaming-product-redcliffe-rsl-card-based-trial-august-2008

Schrans, T., Grace, J., & Schellinck, T. (2004). *2003 NS VL Responsible Gaming Features Evaluation: Final report*. Halifax, NS: Nova Scotia Gaming Corporation.

Schuler, A., Ferentzy, P., Turner, N. E., Skinner, W., McIsaac, K. E., Ziegler, C. P., & Matheson, F. I. (2016). Gamblers Anonymous as a Recovery Pathway: A Scoping Review. *Journal of Gambling Studies*, *32*(4), 1261–1278. doi: 10.1007/s10899-016-9596-8

Schüll, N. (2012). *Addiction by Design. Machine Gambling in Las Vegas*. Princeton: Princeton University Press.

Schwartz, D. (2006). *Roll the Bones: The History of Gambling*. New York: Gotham Books.

Scull S., & Woolcock G. (2005). Problem Gambling in Non-English Speaking Background Communities in Queensland, Australia: A Qualitative Exploration, *International Gambling Studies*, *5*(1), 29–44.

Sender, H. (2014). Illegal Sports Betting Around the World. *International Business Times*, May, 15 http://www.ibtimes.com/illegal-sports-betting-around-world-1584974

Sévigny, S., Cloutier, M., Pelletier, M.-F., & Ladouceur, R. (2005). Internet Gambling: Misleading Payout Rates During the "Demo" Period. *Computers in Human Behavior*, *21*(1), 153–158. https://doi.org/10.1016/j.chb.2004.02.017

Shaffer, H. (2005). From Disabling to Enabling the Public Interest: Natural Transitions from Gambling Exposure to Adaptation and Self-Regulation. *Addiction, 100*(9), 1227–1230.

Shaffer, H. J., & Hall, M. N. (1996). Estimating the Prevalence of Adolescent Gambling Disorders: A Quantitative Synthesis and Guide Toward Standard Gambling Nomenclature. *Journal of Gambling Studies, 12*(2), 193–214.

Shaffer, H. & Korn, D. (2002). Gambling and Related Mental Disorders: A Public Health Analysis. *Annual Review of Public Health 23*, 171–212.

Shaffer, H., Vander Bilt, J., & Hall, M. N. (1997). *Estimating the Prevalence of Disordered Gambling Behavior in the United States and Canada: A meta-analysis.* Harvard Medical School.

Sharman, S., Dreyer, J., Aitken, M., Clark, L., & Bowden-Jones, H. (2015). Rates of Problematic Gambling in a British Homeless Sample: A Preliminary Study. *Journal of Gambling Studies, 31*(2), 525–532.

Sharp, C., Dellis, A., Hofmeyr, A., Kincaid, H., & Ross, D. (2015). First Evidence of Comorbidity of Problem Gambling and Other Psychiatric Problems in a Representative Urban Sample of South Africa. *Journal of Gambling Studies, 31*(3), 679–694.

Sharpe, L., Walker, M., Coughlan, M., Enersen, K., & Blaszczynski, A. (2005). Structural Changes to Electronic Gaming Machines as Effective Harm Minimization Strategies for Non-Problem and Problem Gamblers. *Journal of Gambling Studies, 21*(4), 503–520. doi: 10.1007/s10899-005-5560-8

Shepel, Y. (2007). Azartnye Igry kak Instrument Razrusheniya Obschestva [Gambling as an instrument of societal destruction]. *Vlast, 7*, 51–65.

Sherman, M. (2017). Justices to Review New Jersey Bid for Legal Sports Betting. *Associated Press* June, 27.

Skog, O. J. (2001). Commentary on Gmel & Rehm's Interpretation of the Theory of Collectivity of Drinking Culture. *Drug and Alcohol Review, 20*(3), 325–331.

Skog, O. J. (1985). The Collectivity of Drinking Cultures: A Theory of the Distribution of Alcohol Consumption. *Addiction, 80*(1), 83–99.

Skog, O. J., & Duckert, F. (1993). The Development of Alcoholics' and Heavy Drinkers' Consumption: A Longitudinal Study. *Journal of Studies on Alcohol, 54*(2), 178–188.

Slutske, W. S., Jackson, K. M., & Sher, K. J. (2003). The Natural History of Problem Gambling from Age 18 to 29. *Journal of Abnormal Psychology, 112*(2), 263.

Smith, G. (2014). The Nature and Scope of Gambling in Canada. *Addiction, 109*, 706–710.

Smith, G., Wynne, H., & Hartnagel, T. (2003). *Examining Police Records to Assess Gambling Impacts: A Study of Gambling-Related Crime in the City of Edmonton.* Edmonton: Alberta Gaming Research Institute.

Smith, J. (2000). Gambling Taxation: Public Equity in the Gambling Business. *Australian Economic Review, 33*(2), 120–144.

Sobrun-Maharaj, A., Rossen, F., & Wong, M. A. S. K. (2012*). The Impact of Gambling and Problem Gambling on Asian Families and Communities in New Zealand.* Report for the Ministry of Health. Auckland: Auckland UniServices Ltd. https://www.health.govt.nz/system/files/documents/pages/impact-gambling-asian-communities.pdf

South Australian Centre for Economic Studies (2008). *Social and Economic Impact Study into Gambling in Tasmania.* Report commissioned by Department of Treasury and Finance, Tasmania.

South Australian Centre for Economic Studies (2005). *Study of the Impact of Caps on Electronic Gaming Machines: Final Report.* http://www.justice.vic.gov.au

South Australian Centre for Economic Studies (2003). *Evaluation of self-exclusion programs and harm minimisation measures. Report A.* http://www.adelaide.edu.au/saces/docs/publications-reports/completereportselfexclusiona.pdf

Spapens, T. (2014). Illegal Gambling, in L. Paoli ed., *The Oxford Handbook of Organized Crime.* Oxford: Oxford University Press, 402–418.

Spapens, T. (2012). Gambling: Legal, in M. Beare, ed., *Encyclopedia of Transnational Crime and Justice.* London: Sage, 156–157.

Spapens T. (2008a). Crime Problems Related to Gambling: An Overview, in A. Spapens, A. Littler, & C. J. Fijnaut eds., *Crime, Addiction and the Regulation of Gambling.* Leiden: Martinus Nijhoff Publishers, 19–54.

Spapens, T. (2008b). Regulating the Illegal Gambling Markets: The Case of Illegal Casinos in the Netherlands, in A. Spapens, A. Littler, & C. J. Fijnaut eds., *Crime, Addiction and the Regulation of Gambling.* Leiden: Martinus Nijhoff Publishers, 93–107.

Specker, S.M., Carlson, G.A., Christenson, G.A., & Marcotte, M. (1995). Impulse Control Disorders and Attention Deficit Disorder in Pathological Gamblers. *Annals of Clinical Psychiatry, 7*(4), 175–179.

Spenwyn, J., Barrett, D., & Griffiths, M. (2010). The Role of Light and Music in Gambling Behaviour: An Empirical Pilot Study. *International Journal of Mental Health and Addiction, 8*(1), 107–118. doi: 10.1007/s11469-009-9226-0

Stevens, M., & Bailie, R. (2012). Gambling, Housing Conditions, Community Contexts and Child Health in Remote Indigenous Communities in the Northern Territory, Australia. *BMC Public Health, 12*(1), 377.

Stewart, M., Wohl., M. (2013). Pop-Up Messages, Dissociation, and Craving: How Monetary Limit Reminders Facilitate Adherence in a Session of Slot Machine Gambling. *Psychology of Addictive Behaviors, 27*(1), 268–273. http://dx.doi.org/10.1037/a0029882

Stewart, R. M., & Brown, R. I. (1988). An Outcome Study of Gamblers Anonymous. *The British Journal of Psychiatry, 152*(2), 284–288. doi: 10.1192/bjp.152.2.284

Stinchfield, R. D., & Winters, K. C. (1996). *Treatment Effectiveness of Six State-Supported Compulsive Gambling Treatment Programs in Minnesota.* Minneapolis: Department of Psychiatry, University of Minnesota.

Storer, J., Abbott, M., & Stubbs, J. (2009). Access or Adaptation? A Meta-Analysis of Surveys of Problem Gambling Prevalence in Australia and New Zealand with Respect to Concentration of Electronic Gaming Machines. *International Gambling Studies, 9*(3), 225–244.

Stradbrooke, S. (2017). Italy's Online Gambling Market Now Second Largest in Europe. Shared Experiences. https://calvinayre.com/2017/04/12/business/italys-online-gambling-market-second-uk/

Stutz, H. (2014). Gaming Companies Have Lucrative Deals Operating Indian Casinos, *Las Vegas Review-Journal,* January, 26. https://www.reviewjournal.com/business/gaming-companies-have-lucrative-deals-operating-indian-casinos/

Stymne, A. (2008). *Motives Behind and Effects of State-Owned Netpoker.* Östersund: Swedish National Institute of Public Health.

Sulkunen, P. (2015). The Images Theory of Addiction. *International Journal of Alcohol and Drug Research, 4*(1), 5–11.

Sulkunen, P. & Rantala, V. (2012). Is Pathological Gambling Also an Addiction and Not Just a Big Problem? *Addiction Research and Theory, 20*(1), 1–10.

Sulkunen, P., & Warsell, L. (2012). Universalism Against Particularism. Kettil Bruun and the Ideological Background of the Total Consumption Model. *Nordic Studies on Alcohol and Drugs, 29*(3), 217–232.

Sullivan, S., & Beer, H. (2003). Smoking and Problem Gambling in NZ: Problem Gamblers' Rates of Smoking Increase When They Gamble. *Health Promotion Journal of Australia, 14*(3), 192–195.

Summers Robinson, S., Honeyman, D. S., & Wattenbarger, J. L. (1997). The Resource Suppression and Redistribution Effects of an Earmarked State Lottery, in W. R. Eadington & J. A. Cornelius eds., *Gambling: Public Policies and the Social Sciences.* Reno: Institute for the Study of Gambling and Commercial Gaming, University of Nevada, 537–560.

Suomi, A., Dowling, N. A., & Jackson, A. C. (2014). Problem Gambling Subtypes Based on Psychological Distress, Alcohol Abuse and Impulsivity. *Addictive Behaviors, 39*(12), 1741–1745.

Svenska Spel (2011). *Svenska Spel Annual Report.* English. https://svenskaspel.se/img/omsvs/2011/engl/pdf/svspel_ar_2011-en.pdf

Szczyrba, Z., Fiedor, D., & Smolová, I. (2016). Gamblerization of Post-Communist Society in Central Europe. 16th International Conference on Gambling & Risk Taking, June 8, 2016, Las Vegas. Audio recording available at: http://digitalscholarship.unlv.edu/gaming_institute/2016/June8/15/

Szczyrba, Z., Mravčík, V., Fiedor, D., Černý, J., & Smolová, I. (2015). Gambling in the Czech Republic. *Addiction, 110*(7), 1076–1081. doi: 10.1111/add.12884

Tabri, N., Dupuis, D. R., Kim, H. S., & Wohl, M. J. (2015). Economic Mobility Moderates the Effect of Relative Deprivation on Financial Gambling Motives and Disordered Gambling. *International Gambling Studies, 15*(2), 309–323.

Tammi, T. (2008). Yksinoikeus Peleihin, Yksinoikeus Ongelmiin? Miksirahapeliongelmasta Tuli Yhteiskunnallinen Huolenaihe. *Yhteiskuntapolitiikka, 73*(2), 176–184.

Tammi, T., Castrén, S., & Lintonen, T. (2015). Gambling in Finland: Problem Gambling in the Context of a National Monopoly in the European Union. *Addiction, 110*(5), 746–750. doi: 10.1111/add.12877

Tan, A. K., & Yen, S. T. et al. (2010). Socio-Demographic Determinants of Gambling Participation and Expenditures: Evidence from Malaysia. *International Journal of Consumer* Studies, *34*(3), 316–325.

Tarasov, O. (2010). *Azartnye igry v Sovetskom Soyuze.* [Gambling in the Soviet Union] http://statehistory.ru/973/Azartnye-igry-v-Sovetskom-Soyuze/

Tavares, H. (2014). Gambling in Brazil: A Call for an Open Debate. *Addiction, 109*(12), 1972–1976. doi: 10.1111/add.12560

Taylor, B., Irving, H. M., Kanteres, F., Room, R., Borges, G., Cherpitel, C., ... & Rehm, J. (2010). The More You Drink, the Harder You Fall: A Systematic Review and Meta-Analysis of How Acute Alcohol Consumption and Injury or Collision Risk Increase Together. *Drug and Alcohol Dependence, 110*(1), 108–116.

Teo, P., Mythily, S., Anantha, S., & Winslow, M. (2007). Demographic and Clinical Features of 150 Pathological Gamblers Referred to a Community Addictions Programme. *Annals of the Academy of Medicine, Singapore, 36*(3), 165–168.

Tepperman, L., & Korn, D. (2004). At Home with Gambling: An Exploratory Study. Toronto, ON: Ontario Problem Gambling Research Centre. http://www.gamblingresearch.org/

Thalheimer, R., & Ali, M. M. (2004). The Relationship of Pari-Mutuel Wagering and Casino Gaming to Personal Bankruptcy. *Contemporary Economic Policy*, *22*(3), 420–432.

Thomas, A., Pfeifer, J., Moore, S., Meyer, D., Yap, L., & Armstrong, A. (2013). *Evaluation of the Removal of ATMs from Gaming Venues in Victoria, Australia*.

Thomas, S., Lewis, S., Duong, J., & McLeod, C. (2012). Sports Betting Marketing During Sporting Events: A Stadium and Broadcast Census of Australian Football League Matches. *Australian and New Zealand Journal of Public Health*, *36*(2), 145–152.

Thompson, W. (2010). Gambling in America: *Encyclopedia of History, Issues, and Society* (2nd edn). Santa Barbara: ABC-CLIO.

Thomsen, K. R., Callesen, M. B., Linnet, J., Kringelbach, M. L., & Moller, A. (2009). Severity of Gambling is Associated with Severity of Depressive Symptoms in Pathological Gamblers. *Behavioural Pharmacology*, *20*(5–6), 527–536.

Thomson, G., & Cheng, E. (2013). *Charity Lotteries in Canada: An Examination of Charities Holding Mega Lotteries in Canada*. Charity Intelligence Canada. https://www.charityintelligence.ca/images/2013_lottery_report_web2.pdf

Thon, N., Preuss, U.W., Polzleitner, A., Quantschnig, B., Scholz, H., Kuhberger, A., Bischof, A., Rumpf, H.J., & Wurst, F.M. (2014). Prevalence of Suicide Attempts in Pathological Gamblers in a Nationwide Austrian Treatment Sample. *General Hospital Psychiatry*, *36*(3), 342–346.

Toneatto, T., & Ladoceur, R. (2003). Treatment of Pathological Gambling: A Critical Review of the Literature. *Psychology of Addictive Behaviors*, *17*(4), 284–292. http://dx.doi.org/10.1037/0893-164X.17.4.284

Tong, H. H. Y., & Chim, D., (2013). The Relationship Between Casino Proximity and Problem Gambling. *Asian Journal of Gambling Issues and Public Health 3*(1), 2. http://ajgiph.springeropen.com/articles/10.1186/2195-3007-3-2

Tovar, M.-L., Costes, J.-M., & Eroukmanoff, V. (2013). Les Jeux d'Argent et de Hasard sur Internet en France en 2012. *OFDT*, *85*, 6.

Trimble, M. (2015). Extraterritorial Enforcement of National Laws in Connection with Online Commercial Activity, in J. Rothchild ed., *Research Handbook on Electronic Commerce Law*. Cheltenham, UK and Northampton, Mass., US: Edward Elgar. https://papers.ssrn.com/sol3/papers.cfm?abstract_id=2600925

Trimble, M. (2013). Proposal for an International Convention on Online Gambling, chapter 11, in Pindell, N. & Cabot, A., eds. *Regulating Internet Gaming: Challenges and Opportunities*. Las Vegas: UNLV Gaming Press. http://scholars.law.unlv.edu/cgi/viewcontent.cgi?article=1715&context=facpub

Trucy, F. (2006). *L'Evolution des Jeux de Hasard et d'Argent: le Modèle Français à l'Epreuve*. Sénat: Rapport d'information n° 58.

Tsytsarev, S. (2008). *Problem Gambling in Russia*. Paper presented at the 7th European conference on gambling studies and policy issues, Nova Gorica. http://www.easg.org/media/file/conferences/novagorica2008/thursday/1400-ses2/tsytsarev_sergei.pdf

Tsytsarev, S., & Gilinsky, Y. (2009). Gambling in Russia, in G. Meyer, T. Hayer, & M. Griffiths, eds., *Problem Gaming in Europe: Challenges, Prevention, and Interventions*. New York: Springer, 243–256.

Tu, D., Gray, R. J., & Walton, D. K. (2014). Household Experience of Gambling-Related Harm by Socio-Economic Deprivation in New Zealand: Increases in Inequality between 2008 and 2012. *International Gambling Studies, 14*(2), 330–344.

Turay, S. (2007). *La Française des Jeux:* Jackpot de l'État. Paris: First.

Valentine, G., & Hughes, K. (2010). Ripples in a Pond: The Disclosure to, and Management of, Problem Internet Gambling with/in the Family. *Community, Work & Family, 13*(3), 273–290.

Valleur, M. (2015). Gambling and Gambling-Related Problems in France. *Addiction, 110*(12), 1872–1876. doi: 10.1111/add.12967

Valleur, M. (2008). Le Jeu Comme une Drogue, in M. Fèvre & F. Durand, eds., *Jeux de Hasard et Société*. Paris: L'Harmattan, 59–66.

Vander Bilt J., & Franklin J. (2003). Gambling in a Familial Context, in H. Shaffer, M. N. Hall, J. Vander Bilt & E. M. George, eds., *Futures at Stake: Youth, Gambling, and Society*. Reno: University of Nevada Press, 100–125.

Vasiliadis, S., Jackson, A., Christenson, D. & Francis, K. (2013). Physical Accessibility of Gaming Opportunities and its Relationship to Gaming Involvement and Problem Gambling: A Systematic Review. *Journal of Gambling Issues, 28*, 1–46.

Vasiliev, P., & Bernhard, B. (2012). Prohibitions and Policy in the Global Gambling Industry: A Genealogy and Media Content Analysis of Gaming Restrictions in Contemporary Russia. *UNLV Gaming Research & Review Journal, 15*(1), 71–86.

Velleman, R., Cousins, J., & Orford, J. (2015). Effects of Gambling on the Family, in H. Jones & G. Sanju, eds., *A Clinician's Guide to Working with Problem Gamblers Bowden*. New York: Routledge, 90–103.

Victorian Competition & Efficiency Commission (2012). *Counting the cost: Inquiry into the costs of problem gambling*. Victorian Competition and Efficiency Commission.

Victorian Responsible Gambling Foundation (2014). Victorian Government Announces Agreement with Crown over EGM Levy and VIP Taxes—Bill Introduced. October, 14.

Villeneuve, J., & Pasquier, M. (2011). *Le Tactilo: Au Coeur du Débat sur la Régulation des Jeux de Hasard et d'Argent*. Lausanne: Institut de hautes études en administration publique.

Vitaro, F., Wanner, B., Brendgen, M., & Tremblay, R. E. (2008). Offspring of Parents with Gambling Problems: Adjustment Problems and Explanatory Mechanisms. *Journal of Gambling Studies, 24*(4), 535–553.

Vlaemminck, P., Verbecke, R., Guzik, B., & Van den Bon, J. (2017). Gambling and European law. The Gambling Law Review, no. 2. https://thelawreviews.co.uk/edition/the-gambling-law-review-edition-2/1144045/gambling-and-european-law

Volberg, R.A., & Abbott, M. (2005). *Report Concerning the Regulation of VLTs in Norway*. Northampton MA: Gemini Research.

Volberg, R.A., Gupta, R., Griffiths, M. D., Ólason, D. T., & Delfabbro, P. (2010). An International Perspective on Youth Gambling Prevalence Studies. *International Journal of Adolescent Medicine and Health, 22*(1), 3–38.

Volberg, R.A., Toce, M. T., & Gerstein, D. R. (1999). From Back Room to Living Room: Changing Attitudes Toward Gambling. *Public Perspective, 10*(5), 8–13.

Volberg, R.A., & Wray, M. (2007). Legal Gambling and Problem Gambling as Mechanisms of Social Domination? Some Considerations for Future Research. *American Behavioral Scientist, 51*(1), 56–85.

Walker, D. (2007). Problems in Quantifying the Social Costs and Benefits of Gambling. *American Journal of Economics and Sociology, 66*(3), 609–645.

Walker, D., & Calcagno, P. (2013). Casinos and Political Corruption in the United States: A Granger Causality Analysis. *Applied Economics, 45*(34), 4781–4795.

Walker, D., & Jackson, J. (2011). The Effect of Legalized Gambling on State Goverment Revenue. *Contemporary Economic Policy, 29*(1), 101–114. doi: 10.1111/j.1465-7287.2010.00198.x

Walker, M., & Dickerson, M. (1996). The Prevalence of Problem and Pathological Gambling: A Critical Analysis. *Journal of Gambling Studies, 12*(2), 233–249.

Walker, S. E., Abbott, M. W., & Gray, R. J. (2012). Knowledge, Views and Experiences of Gambling and Gambling-Related Harms in Different Ethnic and Socio-Economic Groups in New Zealand. *Australian New Zealand Journal Public Health, 36*(2), 153–159.

Wall, M., Peter, M., You, R., Mavoa, S., & Witten, K. (2010). *Problem Gambling Research: A Study of Community Level Harm from Gambling.* Phase one Final Report: Report to Ministry of Health. Auckland, New Zealand, Centre for Social and Health Outcomes Research and Evaluation & Te Ropu Whariki.

Walsh et al. (1991). Randomized Trial of Treatment Options for Alcohol-Abusing Workers. *The New England Journal of Medicine, 325,* 775–782.

Wang, P., & Antonopoulos, G. A. (2015). Organized Crime and Illegal Gambling: How Do Illegal Gambling Enterprises Respond to the Challenges Posed by Their Illegality in China? *Australian & New Zealand Journal of Criminology, 49*(2), 258–280.

Wardle, H., Keily, R., Astbury, G., & Reith, G. (2014). Risky Places? Mapping Gambling Machine Density and Socio-Economic Deprivation. *Journal of Gambling Studies, 30*(1), 201–212.

Wardle, H., Moody, A., Griffiths, M., Orford, J., & Volberg, R. (2011a). Defining the Online Gambler and Patterns of Behaviour Integration: Evidence from the British Gambling Prevalence Survey 2010. *International Gambling Studies, 11*(83), 339–356.

Wardle, H., Moody, A., Spence, S., Orford, J., Volberg, R., Jotangia, D., Griffiths, M., Hussey, D., & Dobbie, F. (2011b). *British Gambling Prevalence Survey 2010.* National Centre for Social Research.

Warfield, B. (2008). *Gambling Motivated Fraud in Australia 1998–2007.* Warfield & Associates. https://warfield.com.au/wp-content/uploads/2015/12/pub5.pdf

Warren, J. (2013). *Gambling, the State and Society in Thailand. 1800–1945.* London and NY: Routledge.

Weinstock, J., Ledgerwood, D. M., & Petry, N. M. (2007). Association Between Post Treatment Gambling Behavior and Harm in Pathological Gamblers. *Psychology of Addictive Behaviors, 21,* 185–193.

Welte, J. W., Barnes, G. M., Tidwell, M. C. O., Hoffman, J. H., & Wieczorek, W. F. (2015). Gambling and Problem Gambling in the United States: Changes between 1999 and 2013. *Journal of Gambling Studies, 31*(3), 695–715.

Welte, J. W., Barnes, G. M., Wieczorek, W. F., Tidwell, M. C. O., & Hoffman, J. H. (2007). Type of Gambling and Availability as Risk Factors for Problem Gambling: A Tobit Regression Analysis by Age and Gender. *International Gambling Studies, 7*(2), 183–198.

Welte, J. W., Barnes, G. M., Wieczorek, W. F., Tidwell, M-C., & Parker, J. (2002). Gambling Participation in the US—Results from a National Survey. *Journal of Gambling Studies, 18*(4), 313–337.

Welte, J., Barnes, G., Wieczorek, W., Tidwell, M-C., & Parker, J. (2001). Alcohol and Gambling Pathology among U.S. Adults: Prevalence, Demographic Patterns and Comorbidity. *Journal of Studies on Alcohol, 62*, 706–712.

Welte, J., Wieczorek, W., Barnes, G., Tidwell, M-C., & Hoffman, J. (2004a). The Relationship of Ecological and Geographic Factors to Gambling Behaviour and Pathology. *Journal of Gambling Studies, 20*(4), 405–423.

Welte, J., Wieczorek, W., Tidwell, M-C. & Parker, J. (2004b). Risk Factors for Pathological Gambling. *Addictive Behaviors, 29*, 323–335.

Wenzel, M., McMillan, J., Marshall, D., & Ahmed, E. (2004). Validation of the Victorian Gambling Screen. GRP Report No. 7, Centre for Gambling Research, Canberra, Australia. https://openresearch-repository.anu.edu.au/bitstream/1885/45190/3/WholeVicGamScr_03.pdf

Wenzel, H. G., Øren, A., & Bakken, I. J. (2008). Gambling problems in the Family—A Stratified Probability Sample Study of Prevalence and Reported Consequences. *BMC Public Health, 8*(1), 412.

Westfelt, L. (2006). *Statliga kasinon i Sundsvall och Malmö: Forväntningar, Erfarenheter, Attityder, Spelande och Spelproblem Fore Etablingeringen Samt Ett År och Tre År Efter* [State casinos in Sundsvall and Malmö: Expectations, experiences, attitudes to gambling and problem gambling before the establishment and one year and three years after]. Research Report No. 3. SoRAD, Stockholm University.

Wheeler, B. W., Rigby, J. E., & Huriwai, T. (2006). Pokies and Poverty: Problem Gambling Risk Factor Geography in New Zealand. *Health & Place, 12*, 86–96.

Wheeler, S. A., Round, D. K., & Wilson, J. K. (2010). The Relationship Between Crime and Electronic Gaming Expenditure: Evidence from Victoria, Australia. *Journal of Quantitative Criminology, 27*(3), 315–338.

Wiebe J. & Lipton M. D. (2008). *An Overview of Internet Gambling Regulations*. Ontario Problem Gambling Research Centre, Canada.

Wiggins, L., Nower, L., Mayers, R. S., & Peterson, N. A. (2010). A Geospatial Statistical Analysis of the Density of Lottery Outlets within Ethnically Concentrated Neighborhoods. *Journal of Community Psychology, 38*(4), 486–496.

Williams, R. J., Belanger, Y. D., & Arthur, J. N. (2011a). *Gambling in Alberta: History, Current Status and Socioeconomic Impacts*. Alberta Gaming Research Institute.

Williams, R. J., Lee, C. K., & Back, K. J. (2013). The Prevalence and Nature of Gambling and Problem Gambling in South Korea. *Social Psychiatry and Psychiatric Epidemiology, 48*(5), 821–834.

Williams R. J., Rehm, J., & Stevens, R. M. G. (2011b). *The Social and Economic Impacts of Gambling*. Final Report to the Canadian Interprovincial Consortium for Gambling Research.

Williams, R. J., Royston, J., & Hagen, B. F. (2005). Gambling and Problem Gambling Within Forensic Populations: A Review of the Literature. *Criminal Justice and Behavior, 32*(6), 665–689.

Williams, R. J., & Volberg, R. A. (2014). The Classification Accuracy of Four Problem Gambling Assessment Instruments in Population Research. *International Gambling Studies, 14*(1), 15–28.

Williams, R. J., & Volberg, R. A. (2010). *Best Practices in the Population Assessment of Problem Gambling*. Faculty of Health Sciences. https://www.uleth.ca/dspace/bitstream/handle/10133/1259/2010-BP-OPGRC.pdf?sequence=1&isAllowed=y

Williams R. J., Volberg R. A., Stevens R. M. G. (2012a). *The Population Prevalence of Problem Gambling: Methodological Influences, Standardized Rates, Jurisdictional Differences, and Worldwide Trends.* Ontario Problem Gambling Research Centre.

Williams, R. J., West, B. L., & Simpson, R. I. (2012b). *Prevention of Problem Gambling: A Comprehensive Review of the Evidence and Identified Best Practices.* Ontario Problem Gambling Research Centre and the Ontario Ministry of Health and Long Term Care.

Williams, R. J., & Wood, R. T. (2004). The Proportion of Gaming Revenue Derived from Problem Gamblers: Examining the Issues in a Canadian Context. *Analyses of Social Issues and Public Policy*, 4(1), 33–45.

Williams, R. J., Wood, R. T., & Parke, J. (2012c). *Routledge International Handbook of Internet Gambling.* Oxford: Routledge.

Wilson, D. H., Gilliland, J., Ross, N. A., Derevensky, J., & Gupta, R. (2006). Video Lottery Terminal Access and Gambling Among High School Students in Montreal. *Canadian Journal of Public Health/Revue Canadienne de Santeé Publique*, 202–206.

Wolfson, S. & Case, G. (2000). The Effects of Sound and Colour on Responses to a Computer Game. *Interacting with Computers*, 13(2), 183–192. https://www.sciencedirect.com/science/article/pii/S0953543800000370

Wong P. W., Chan W. S., Conwell Y., Conner K. R., Yip P. S. (2010a). A Psychological Autopsy Study of Pathological Gamblers Who Died by Suicide. *Journal of Affective Disorders*, 120(1), 213–216.

Wong P. W., Cheung D. Y., Conner K. R., Conwell Y., Yip P. S. (2010b). Gambling and Completed Suicide in Hong Kong: A Review of Coroner Court Files. *Primary Care Companion to the Journal of Clinical Psychiatry*, 12(6), e1–7.

Wong, P. W., Kwok, N. C., Tang, J. Y., Blaszczynski, A., & Tse, S. (2014). Suicidal Ideation and Familicidal-Suicidal Ideation Among Individuals Presenting to Problem Gambling Services: A Retrospective Data Analysis. *Crisis: The Journal of Crisis Intervention and Suicide Prevention*, 35(4), 219–232.

Wood, R. T. A., & Griffiths, M. D. (2007). A Qualitative Investigation of Problem Gambling as an Escape-Based Coping Strategy. *Psychology and Psychotherapy: Theory, Research and Practice*, 80(1), 107–125.

Wood, R. T., Williams, R. J., & Lawton, P. (2007). Why do Internet Gamblers Prefer Online Versus Land-Based Venues? *Journal of Gambling Issues*, 20, 235–250. http://hdl.handle.net/10133/375

Wood, R., & Wohl, M. (2015). Assessing the Effectiveness of a Responsible Gambling Behavioural Feedback Tool for Reducing the Gambling Expenditure of At-Risk Players. *International Gambling Studies*, 15(2), 324–339. http://dx.doi.org/10.1080/14459795.2015.1049191

Woolley, R. & Livingstone, C. (2010). Into the Zone. Innovating in the Australian Poker Machine Industry, in S. Kingma ed., *Cultural Perspectives on Gambling Organizations.* New York: Routledge, 38–63.

Woolley, R., Livingstone, C., Harrigan, K., & Rintoul, A. (2013). House Edge: Hold Percentage and the Cost of EGM Gambling. *International Gambling Studies*, 13(3), 388–402.

World Bank (2017). *Population, total.* http://data.worldbank.org/indicator/SP.POP.TOTL

World Health Organization (2008). *Closing the Gap in a Generation. Health Equity Through Action on the Social Determinants of Health.* Final Report of the Commission on Social Determinants of Health. Geneva: World Health Organization.

World Health Organization (1993). *The ICD10 Classification of Mental and Behavioural Disorders: Diagnostic Criteria for Research.* Geneva: World Health Organization.

World Health Organization (2014). *Global Status Report on Alcohol and Health, 2014.* Management of Substance Abuse Unit. Geneva: World Health Organization.

Worthington, A. C. (2001). Implicit Finance in Gambling Expenditures: Australian Evidence on Socioeconomic and Demographic Tax Incidence. *Public Finance Review, 29*(4), 326–342.

Wray M., Miller, M., Gurvey, J., Carroll, J., & Kawachi, I. (2008). Leaving Las Vegas: Exposure to Las Vegas and Risk of Suicide. *Social Science & Medicine, 67*(11), 1882–1888.

Wynne, H. J. (2002). *Gambling and Problem Gambling in Saskatchewan. Final Report.* Canadian Centre on Substance Abuse. https://prism.ucalgary.ca/handle/1880/47571

Wynne, H. J., & Stinchfield, R. (2004). *Evaluating VLT responsible gaming features and interventions in Alberta.* Prepared for the Alberta Gaming and Liquor Commission.

Youn, S., Faber, R. J., & Shah, D. V. (2000). Restricting Gambling Advertising and the Third-Person Effect. *Psychology and Marketing, 17*(7), 633–649. https://pdfs.semanticscholar.org/fc3b/0c2021ba28911e8d2930dd58834ca8b291c7.pdf

Young, M., Markham, F., & Doran, B. (2012). Too Close to Home? The Relationship Between Residential Distance to Venue and Gambling Outcomes. *International Gambling Studies, 12*(2), 257–273.

Young, M., Wohl, M., Matheson, K., Baumann, S., & Anisman, H. (2008). The Desire to Gamble: The Influence of Outcomes on the Priming Effects of a Gambling Episode. *Journal of Gambling Studies, 24*(3), 275–293. doi: 10.1007/s10899-008-9093-9

Index

Note: figures, boxes, and tables are indicated by *f, b,* and *t* following the page number.